TAMING THE BLACK DOG

Revised Edition

BEV AISBETT

HarperCollins*Publishers*

Workshop and lecture information,
and other anxiety resources:
www.bevaisbettartofanxiety.com

HarperCollins*Publishers*
First published in Australia in 2000
This edition published in 2019
by HarperCollins*Publishers* Australia Pty Limited
ABN 36 009 913 517
harpercollins.com.au

HarperCollins*Publishers*
Level 13, 201 Elizabeth Street, Sydney NSW 2000, Australia
Unit D1, 63 Apollo Drive, Rosedale, Auckland 0632, New Zealand
A 53, Sector 57, Noida, UP, India
1 London Bridge Street, London, SE1 9GF, United Kingdom
Bay Adelaide Centre, East Tower, 22 Adelaide Street West, 41st floor, Toronto,
    Ontario M5H 4E3, Canada
195 Broadway, New York NY 10007, USA

A catalogue record for this book is available from the National Library of Australia

ISBN 978 1 4607 5696 6 (paperback)
ISBN 978 1 4607 1073 9 (ebook)

Cover design by Hazel Lam, HarperCollins Design Studio
Cover illustration by Bev Aisbett
Printed and bound in Australia by McPherson's Printing Group
The papers used by HarperCollins in the manufacture of this book are a natural,
recyclable product made from wood grown in sustainable plantation forests. The fibre
source and manufacturing processes meet recognised international environmental
standards, and carry certification.

*To Grace, my daughter — who taught me
that too many tears would only
weigh down her wings*

ABOUT THE AUTHOR

Bev Aisbett is the author of highly regarded self-help books — *Living with IT, I Love Me, Get Over IT* and most recently *30 Days 30 Ways to Overcome Anxiety* — which have now helped thousands of people throughout Australia and overseas attain recovery from the crippling effects of anxiety.

For the past twenty-five years, she has conducted the 'Working with IT' workshops — an extensive program aimed to further assist sufferers towards not only recovery from anxiety, but also greater independence, freedom and self-esteem in all areas of their lives.

A past sufferer of both anxiety and depression, Bev now brings her own experience, learning and wisdom to the assistance of people suffering from one of the greatest challenges of modern life — depression — through this book, *Taming the Black Dog*.

Contents

INTRODUCTION
(2000 edition)

I haven't had a very easy life. Like you, I have had a lot of losses and endured a lot of pain.

Sometimes, even now, I will surrender to pain and I will spend a day or two in the miserable company of the Black Dog — DEPRESSION.

I allow him to seduce me, for he offers me the temptation of giving up, of saying 'Too Hard'. He extends to me the luxury of being absolved of all responsibility to address, repair or change my life.

I can even be enticed into thinking that this retreat from life is a kind of relief, a kind of solution, a kind of sanctuary from life.

I can be fooled into thinking that this constitutes a justified protest at the unfairness of the world — 'See how you've hurt me? Aren't you sorry?' — as if this will change anything.

I can even believe that the Black Dog comes and goes as he pleases — that I have no choice and no control over when he will visit or how long he will stay.

But these days, I can only convince myself of this for a short time, for I have looked into the eyes of the Black Dog and seen what he is made of — ILLUSIONS.

And an illusion, once exposed, can never really exert the same power again.

I now know that if the Black Dog comes, I have opened the door and let him in; and if and when the Black Dog goes it is I who have sent him away.

This little book is aimed to make you, too, master of the Black Dog, instead of his victim.

It will show you his tricks and how to take control. This takes time. Sometimes he is very stubborn, but in the end, he just needs someone to show him the way.

It's *your* life, not his. Claim it back — it's precious. There *is* hope, and there is a way, even though you may not see it. You just haven't got to that bit, yet. WAIT ...

This, too, will pass.

NEW INTRODUCTION
(2019 edition)

Depression is a tough nut to crack. In my experience, it is easier to calm someone down from anxiety than it is to coax someone from the dense, heavy cloud of inertia that comes with depression.

Above all, depression is very stubborn. Or am I talking about people with depression? I mean no disrespect, but people with depression can be very resistant to the idea of being helped to overcome their malaise, pessimistic world view and depression.

I know this from personal experience. Depression is very compelling and, in many ways, very addictive.

I've never been a big fan of the idea that we're stuck with anything! I think in a majority of cases, we get ourselves stuck and, even if we find ourselves stuck through extenuating circumstances, we tend to *keep* ourselves stuck. And we have a choice to continue to do this or not.

The challenge is in getting someone to the point where they are ready and willing to make the choice to become unstuck and to *keep* making it.

When I write my books — especially this revision — my touchstone is 'What would have got through to me when I was most resistant?'

For sure, apart from a few occasions, it wasn't when someone was patting my hand. As loving and as soothing as that may have been, it was not going to encourage me to step out of my sadness as much as hold on to it.

What made the difference was someone calling on me to be the best version of myself; someone who refused to join me in justifying my limitations.

They showed me that I was short-changing myself and that no-one was meant to live this miserable, shrunken, collapsed way of being.

They showed me I had a choice — I could keep telling the same old. sad story or not; I could define myself by my hurts and losses or not.

That's the choice you need to make. And you will only make it when you realise that you're WORTHY of a whole lot better than this.

And that's the biggest choice you need to make. To recognise that you're worth the effort of putting in the work to be well.

I want you well. This is the work that made — and keeps — me well.

Introducing The Black Dog

The legendary wartime leader, WINSTON CHURCHILL, suffered from DEPRESSION most of his life.

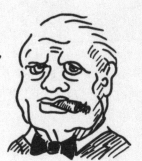

He named his Depression the 'BLACK DOG'.

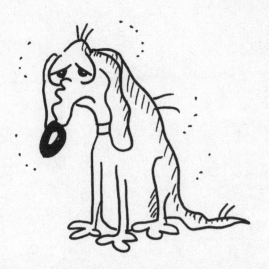

Has the BLACK DOG moved into your life?

Has he TAKEN OVER?

How do you TAME him?

This book is a TRAINING MANUAL to help you TAME YOUR BLACK DOG.

RECOGNISING
THE
BLACK DOG

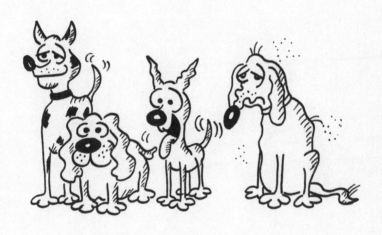

WHEN DEPRESSION
BECOMES A PROBLEM

Most of us feel depressed from time to time. This is usually linked to changes, losses and setbacks that are part of life.

These may include:

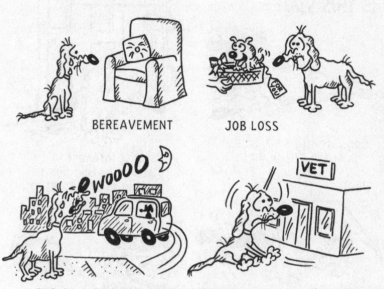

BEREAVEMENT   JOB LOSS

END OF A RELATIONSHIP   PHYSICAL CHANGES/PROBLEMS

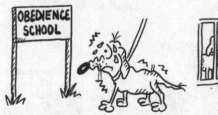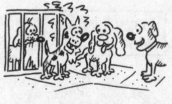

TESTS OF ABILITY OR WORTH   SOCIAL PROBLEMS, ETC.

Depression associated with such life events, though painful, is usually TEMPORARY and lifts once life returns to normal or a reasonable period of grieving has passed.

Depression may be a problem, however, if it is ONGOING and not apparently linked to an OBVIOUS CAUSE.

IS THIS YOU?

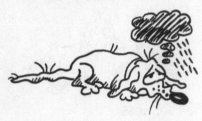

Consistently SAD, BLUE, DOWN IN THE DUMPS?

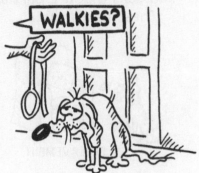

Lost interest in activities you used to find PLEASURABLE?

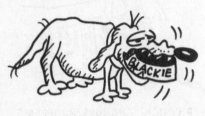

OVEREATING

OR

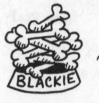

LACK of APPETITE?

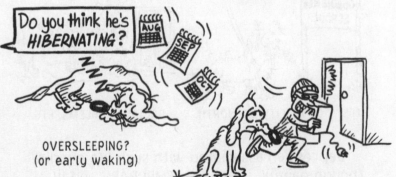

OVERSLEEPING?
(or early waking)

LESS ACTIVE or TALKATIVE than usual?

6

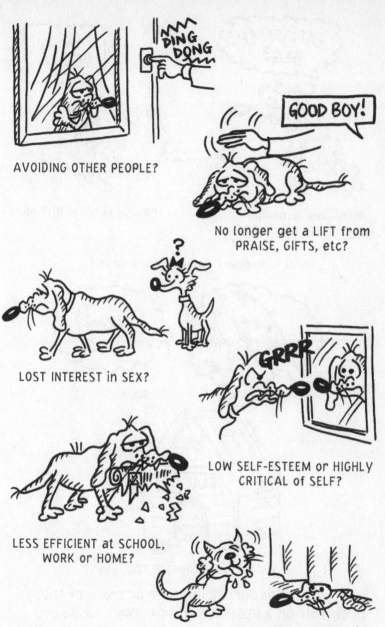

AVOIDING OTHER PEOPLE?

No longer get a LIFT from PRAISE, GIFTS, etc?

LOST INTEREST in SEX?

LOW SELF-ESTEEM or HIGHLY CRITICAL of SELF?

LESS EFFICIENT at SCHOOL, WORK or HOME?

Less able to COPE with EVERYDAY ROUTINES?

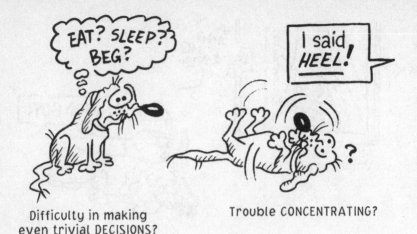

Difficulty in making
even trivial DECISIONS?

Trouble CONCENTRATING?

And sometimes do you find yourself ...

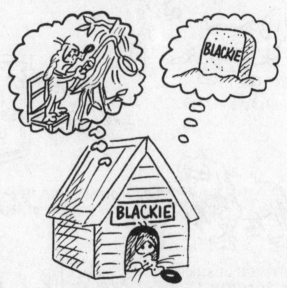

...entertaining MORBID THOUGHTS?

If you are experiencing four or more of these
problems on a REGULAR and ONGOING basis, you
may have a problem with depression which will
require ATTENTION.

2

WHEN THE BLACK DOG MOVES IN

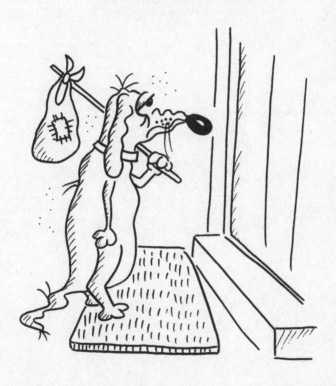

THE SYMPTOMS OF DEPRESSION

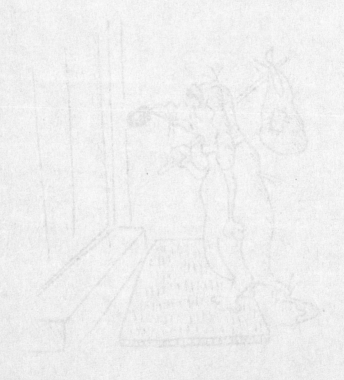

It is very painful living with depression.

The colour seems to drain out of the world.

The nights seem unbearably long.

Nothing seems to bring comfort — not love, concern or sympathy.

You feel alone, even in a group.

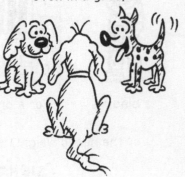

People describe Depression in many different ways, but the most common images are ...

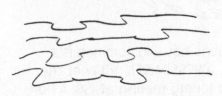

... being lost in a fog

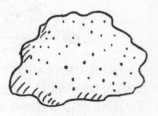

or being pressed down by a great weight.

11

Some describe

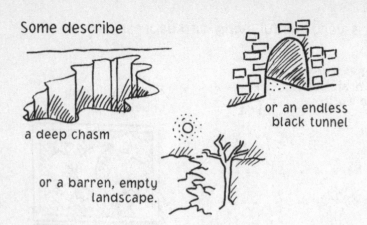

a deep chasm

or an endless
black tunnel

or a barren, empty
landscape.

Sometimes depression may feel like ...

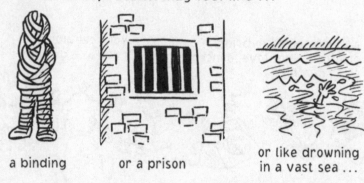

a binding   or a prison   or like drowning
in a vast sea ...

... or the heavy weight, the burden of THE BLACK DOG.

-SIGH-

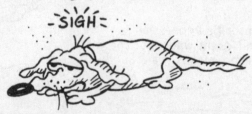

What these descriptions have in common is a
sense of HOPELESSNESS, a PESSIMISTIC VIEW of the
FUTURE and a deep and lonely feeling of ISOLATION.

But ... YOU ARE NOT ALONE!

In fact, the World Health Organisation has even suggested that a staggering 100 MILLION people are depressed at any one time ... a statistic that may not really CHEER YOU UP!!

However, if we examine this figure more closely, it includes ANYONE who has EVER felt a BIT BLUE, to DEEPLY SAD to INCREDIBLY DOWN, LOST or MISERABLE (about 90% of us at some time)!

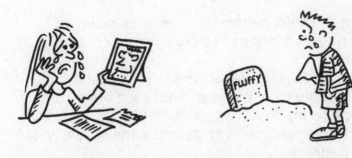

More severe depression, which seriously affects a person's ability to FUNCTION NORMALLY is rated at about 15% of the population.

The CLINICAL TERMS for depression include:

REACTIVE OR SITUATIONAL

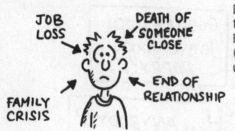

Depression triggered by EXTERNAL events (and therefore usually temporary)

JOB LOSS

DEATH OF SOMEONE CLOSE

END OF RELATIONSHIP

FAMILY CRISIS

ENDOGENOUS

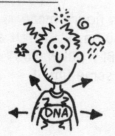

DNA

Depression believed to be triggered by INTERNAL factors, such as genes or biochemical triggers.

ENDOGENOUS depression was once believed to be triggered independently from external events.

These days, however, this is seen as not necessarily true. Both can feed each other.

The terms 'REACTIVE' or 'ENDOGENOUS' are now more commonly used to describe the SEVERITY of the depression.

Causes and triggers are usually a COMBINATION of SEVERAL FACTORS.

These will be explored in following chapters.

Below is a table of different levels of emotional wellbeing. Where do you sit on this scale?

HEALTHY	OUT OF BALANCE	PROBLEMATIC
• Confident	• Need reassurance	• Sense of failure
• Self-worth	• Self-doubt	• Contemptuous of self
• Creative	• Uninspired	• Sees no point in anything
• Loving (to self & others)	• Not generous with affection	• Feeling unloved, unlovable & unloving
• Energy	• Low energy	• Depleted energy
• Interested	• Low enthusiasm	• Uninterested in life
• Sexually active	• Lowered sex drive	• Flat-line sex drive
• Socially involved	• Distant from others	• Withdrawn
• Self-motivated	• Need prodding	• No motivation
• Responsible	• Blames outside factors	• Not looking after self
• Full range of emotions	• Pleasure is compromised	• Feelings of shame, misery and guilt
VERDICT	**VERDICT**	**VERDICT**
OK! STAY!	*TRAINING REQUIRED!*	*UH OH! DOWN!*

3

FLEAS, FUR BALLS
&
MUDDY PAW PRINTS

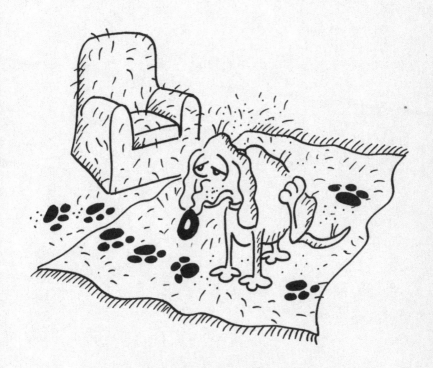

DEPRESSION IN RELATION
TO OTHERS

Depression makes an impact on most areas of your life, but few of these can take such a toll as in your dealings with others during this time.

You may already be experiencing difficulties in your interactions with others.

Some of the problems you may be encountering could include:

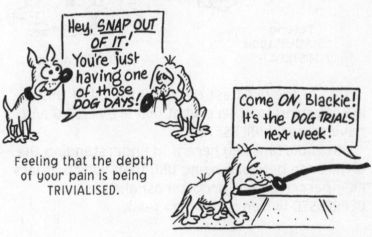

Feeling that the depth of your pain is being TRIVIALISED.

Feeling INADEQUATE and a FAILURE because you ARE depressed.

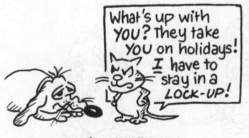

Feeling GUILTY and UNGRATEFUL for being this way.

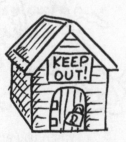

Feeling caught between WANTING to be ALONE and feeling REJECTED if you are.

Cut this *OUT!* I'm *FED UP* with you *MOOCHING AROUND* all *HANGDOG!*

But most of all ...

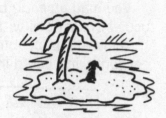

Feeling
MISUNDERSTOOD
or MISTREATED.

Feeling ALONE.

One of the greatest difficulties in all of this is in conveying to others what you are FEELING and having them UNDERSTAND.

An important key here is in understanding the difference between being UNHAPPY (which others may perceive your problem as) and being DEPRESSED (which is how you feel).

WHAT IS THE MAJOR DIFFERENCE?

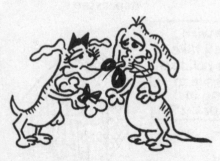

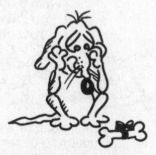

When you are
UNHAPPY you can
SEEK comfort and
ALLOW yourself to
FEEL COMFORTED.

When you are
DEPRESSED, you feel
unable to do EITHER.

This is one of the TRAPS of depressed thinking. The gap between what you are FEELING and what others PERCEIVE can, indeed, contribute greatly to your own sense of ISOLATION.

Some examples:

1. FLATNESS

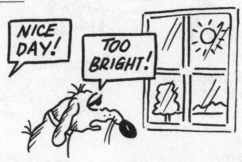

FOR YOU
You no longer find PLEASURE in everyday things. You feel DULLED and FLAT.

FOR OTHERS
Your lack of ENTHUSIASM and NEGATIVITY can detract from others' experience of pleasure, too. They may feel CHEATED.

2. NON-RESPONSIVENESS

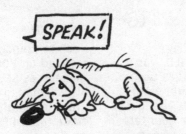

FOR YOU
You find it difficult to COMMUNICATE, because your feelings are CONFUSING and PAINFUL and you LACK ENERGY.

FOR OTHERS
Your reluctance to speak up can make others feel they cannot REACH you. They may feel REJECTED.

3. LETHARGY

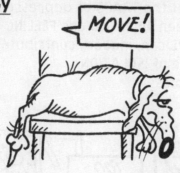

FOR YOU

You feel as though your ENERGY has DISAPPEARED.

And, let's be HONEST ...

FOR OTHERS

Your IMMOBILITY may be seen as LAZINESS or SELF-INDULGENCE.

4. SELF-PITY

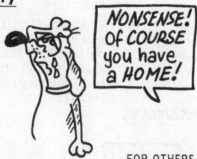

FOR YOU

You feel UNWORTHY, GUILTY and FLAWED. You GRIEVE over the life you have lost (or never had). You've lost HOPE. Yes, you DO feel sorry for yourself and feel you have good reason to.

FOR OTHERS

Your tendency to be focused on YOURSELF may be seen as SELFISH. Others may look at your life and wonder WHAT you have to be DEPRESSED about.

All of these things make it difficult for EITHER PARTY to close the gap by REACHING OUT, but REACHING OUT is CRUCIAL.

WHAT _YOU_ CAN DO

As difficult as it may feel, your recovery can only begin by your making a move towards it.
You need to acknowledge something crucial: NO-ONE ELSE CAN DO THIS FOR YOU. Others can encourage you but ultimately it is YOU taking the steps towards recovery that generate your healing.

This is how it works:

Over here is
DEPRESSION

and over here is
RECOVERY

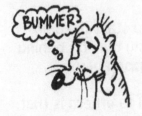

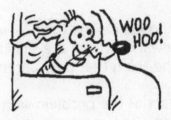

And here you
are right now.

So, which option is
all your attention
focused on?

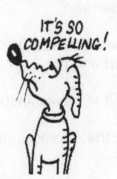

The mistake most people make at this point is thinking they can just stay in this same dynamic and that recovery — or 'rescue' — will somehow just turn up.

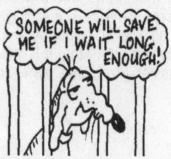

It won't. It's not home-delivered. You must start moving towards it.

And here's the thing — when you start heading towards it, you are simultaneously leaving behind the thing that has currently trapped you.

Part of the problem with regard to others is that, too often, we place our wellbeing in their hands rather than our own.

Think about what caused you to feel so down about yourself and life.

Chances are, it involves another PERSON or PEOPLE.

You may feel that someone hurt you or let you down.

How do you see yourself in relation to others?

Do you constantly compare yourself and find yourself lacking in some way?

Do you need the approval of others to help you feelworthy, loved and secure?

Can you be happy in your own company or do you experience loneliness after even a short time alone?

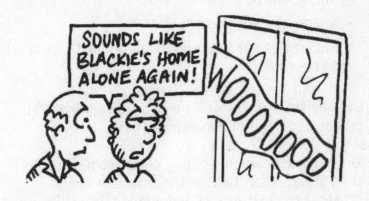

Above all, do you rely on others behaving in a way that pleases you in order for you to maintain your wellbeing?

What if they don't? Do you fall apart?

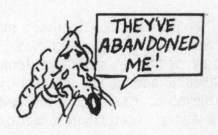

If these things resonate, then perhaps the emphasis on others determining your wellbeing has left you disempowered.

When you look to others to tell you:

- WHO YOU ARE
- WHAT YOU NEED
- WHETHER OR NOT YOU ARE WORTHY
- WHETHER OR NOT YOU ARE LOVABLE
- WHETHER OR NOT YOU ARE STRONG, CAPABLE, OKAY OR EVEN WELL

you are setting yourself up to be disappointed if others don't fulfil your expectations.

These things can only really come from you, and if they aren't, then THAT is the problem — not others, nor what others have 'done' to you.

The relationship you have with YOURSELF is the thing that needs fixing, first and foremost. The rest will follow.

However, REACHING OUT is a vital part of recovery.

When life feels too painful, it may seem like a comfort to shut yourself away, but you then make it harder for yourself to re-emerge. (This is called NUMBING and we will explore that in detail later) Sharing your struggles with another is a crucial first step ih returning to wellbeing.

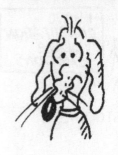

HUH? NOW I'M CONFUSED! YOU'RE SAYING ONLY I CAN HELP MYSELF!?

There is a difference between REACHING OUT and looking to be RESCUED.

REACHING OUT means asking for what you need in order to HELP YOURSELF, instead of hoping that others will just KNOW or will do it FOR you, which keeps you powerless.

Reaching out means you're doing something helpful for yourself. Sharing of yourself with others is worlds apart from NEEDING others to make your life bearable.

FOR YOU:

You DEFINE what your needs are, instead of vague notions

FOR OTHERS:

Others find that they now have PRACTICAL ways to help you.

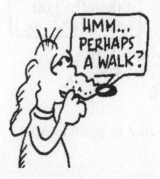

HMM... PERHAPS A WALK?

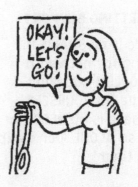

OKAY! LET'S GO!

27

YOU CAN REACH OUT BY:

(A) TALKING IT OUT

Right now, your EMOTIONS
are very STUCK.

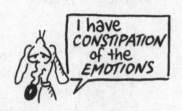

One way to MOVE them
on is to give them an
OUTLET.
Talking to someone FREES UP the STUCKNESS.
It helps THEM understand, too!

(B) GETTING A REALITY CHECK

You are having the experience of being INSIDE
depression looking OUT at life. What you see is
FILTERED through depression. Reality is DISTORTED.

Talking to someone can give you a different
view on the REALITY of the situation.

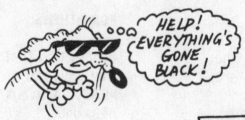

(C) GETTING SUPPORT

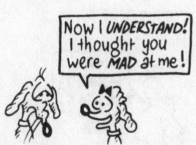

There is no SHAME in
asking for help with
a PROBLEM you can't
handle by YOURSELF.

There is NO NEED to
feel so ALONE. Don't expect people to MIND READ.
TELL them!

IMPORTANT STARTING POINTS:

1. FEELINGS PASS!

Emotions CHANGE.
You are not
actually DEPRESSED
EVERY minute of
EVERY day. It just
FEELS that way.

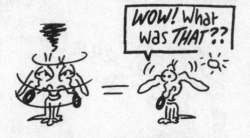

THIS, TOO, WILL PASS!

2. LIFE IS JUST LIFE

HOW IT FEELS DEPENDS
ON HOW YOU FEEL.

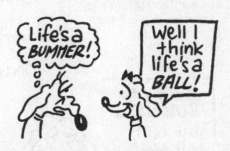

REALITY MAY NOT BE AS IT SEEMS TO BE AT THE MOMENT

3. A PROBLEM SHARED IS A PROBLEM HALVED

☆ Accept that you are NOT
QUITE YOURSELF at
present.

☆ Accept that you may not
have all the ANSWERS.

☆ Accept that you may
need a HAND with this.

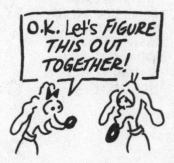

WHAT OTHERS CAN DO—
(SHOW THEM THIS)

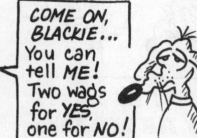

(Once recovered, it's an idea for the sufferer to keep an eye out for these, too.)

1. IDENTIFY THE PROBLEM

As a friend or family member, you may be first to notice early signs of depression. These may include:

☆ Increase in ALCOHOL

☆ IMPULSIVE DECISIONS (e.g. suddenly leaving job)

☆ LETHARGY or LACK OF INTEREST

☆ Increased IRRITABILITY.

COME ON, BLACKIE... You can tell ME! Two wags for YES, one for NO!

Try to encourage the depressed person to open up and give them a safe and non-judgmental space to truly express their feelings.

2. ENCOURAGE COMMUNICATION

The depressed person may be closed up for several reasons:

☆ Feeling ASHAMED or GUILTY

☆ Denying there is a PROBLEM

☆ Not wanting to be 'DOWNER'

☆ Feeling AFRAID to reveal their FEARS, PAIN or EMOTIONS

☆ Fearing REJECTION or RIDICULE.

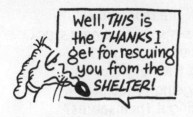

Well, *THIS* is the *THANKS* I get for rescuing you from the *SHELTER!*

Encouragement, understanding, love and patience may be required for some time.

3. BE COMPASSIONATE

No matter whether you think the depressed person is JUSTIFIED in feeling this way, for him/her it is very REAL and OVERWHELMING. He/she cannot just 'SNAP OUT OF IT'.

Remember: YOU ARE WELL. BE PATIENT.

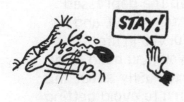

STAY!

Clarify the difference between being helpful and creating a 'VICTIM' mentality.

4. HOLD YOUR PLACE

COMPASSION is one thing but getting caught up in 'RESCUING' will help neither of you move on.

You may end up constantly looking after the depressed person, while they give up on trying to help themselves.

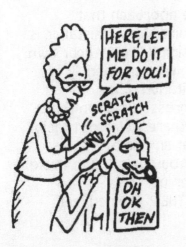

HERE, LET ME DO IT FOR YOU!

SCRATCH SCRATCH

OH OK THEN

5. ENCOURAGE SELF HELP

This is a crucial point as you will need to find a BALANCE between being supportive and taking over responsibility for the depressed person's life, which is and remains their job.

The more you take over, the more you encourage the depressed person to remain stuck.

Think of it this way: if you're constantly jumping the fence to weed the neighbour's garden, they're probably going to let you! Why would they bother doing it themselves?

Above all, treating the depressed person as an invalid is not going to help either of you.

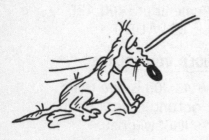

You may need to provide the MOTIVATION that the depressed person lacks at present.

6. KEEP THINGS MOVING

Do whatever you can to keep the depressed person ACTIVE and INVOLVED in life.

You may need to be fairly PUSHY about this.

Try to avoid getting ANGRY, but NOW and THEN you may need to express your FRUSTRATION.

7. BUSINESS AS USUAL

One approach that inspires less resistance is to simply ENJOY your own life, with an open invitation to the depressed person that they are welcome to join in at any time.

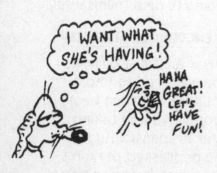

Above all, try to avoid being dragged into the other person's depression. Remember, it's THEIR journey, not yours. Be YOURSELF.

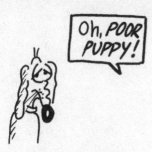

Assessing your
relationship and
aiming to IMPROVE it
can mean CHANGES
all round.

8. ASSESS YOUR PART

Honestly assess whether
your relationship with the
depressed person may
be part of the PROBLEM.
   WITHOUT GUILT ask
yourself:

☆ Do I NEED others to be
   DEPENDENT on me?

☆ Is the relationship
   EQUAL, RESPECTFUL and
   HONEST?

☆ Do I EXPECT a lot from
   others?

☆ Do I tend to TAKE OVER?

☆ Do I treat the depressed
   person as an ADULT or a
   CHILD?

☆ Do I set clear boundaries?

Don't be surprised if your friend's/partner's/family
member's depression brings up some of your own
issues — after all, you are sharing this experience,
especially if you are in an intimate relationship.

   You may need to also do a little soul-searching
(and even seek help) about the part you may be
playing in this dynamic.

   Above all, see this current situation as a
problem requiring a TEAM EFFORT to work
through. ENCOURAGEMENT, FAITH and HOPE from
OTHERS, HONESTY and COMMITTED WORK from YOU,
the sufferer. This book will guide the TEAM.

4

THE BLACK DOG'S OWNER

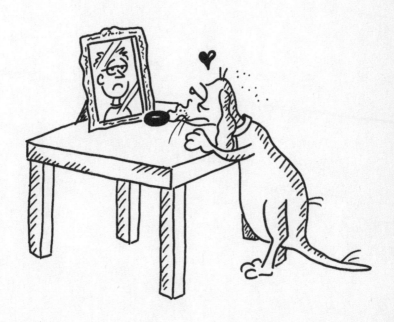

THE ORIGINS OF DEPRESSION

So how did you come to have a BLACK DOG in your life?

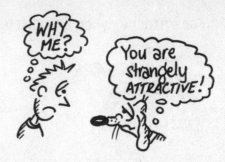

In most cases of EMOTIONAL DISTURBANCE, there is seldom a SINGLE CAUSE but SEVERAL contributing factors that add up over time.

In clinical terms, these are known as —

1. PSYCHODYNAMIC

2. BEHAVIOURAL

3. PHYSICAL

1. PSYCHODYNAMIC WORKS THIS WAY —

In early childhood, BELIEFS about ourselves are created by the way we are treated.

NEGLECT, SHAME, LACK OF LOVE, or even being OVERPROTECTED send strong messages about our worth or ability to handle life.

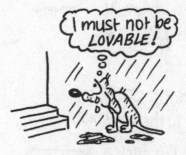

These BELIEFS in turn dictate the way in which we REACT or RESPOND to stressful situations.

For instance, when CRITICISED, you may REACT by:

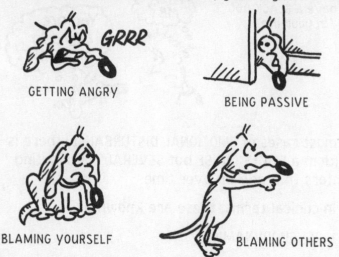

GETTING ANGRY

BEING PASSIVE

BLAMING YOURSELF

BLAMING OTHERS

And these REACTIONS will be fed by certain BELIEFS you hold about YOURSELF.

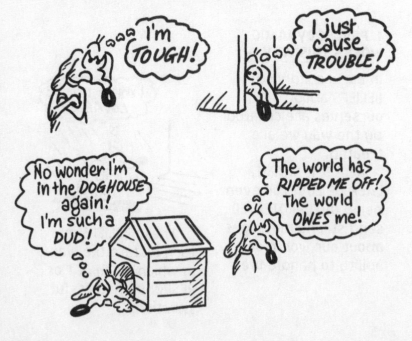

I'm TOUGH!

I just cause TROUBLE!

No wonder I'm in the DOGHOUSE again! I'm such a DUD!

The world has RIPPED ME OFF! The world OWES me!

These REACTIONS and BELIEFS can lead to PATTERNS of behaviour that FURTHER undermine your SELF-ESTEEM as you grow older.

For instance:

Getting ANGRY, BLAMING or being DEFENSIVE with others can make you UNPOPULAR.

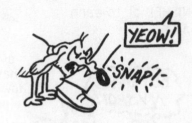

Being PASSIVE may mean that you tend to be OVERLOOKED.

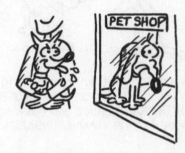

Blaming YOURSELF may mean that you do not gain RESPECT.

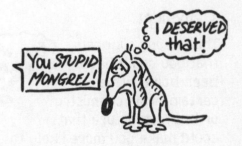

PSYCHODYNAMIC thus refers to the MIND (PSYCHE) affecting BEHAVIOUR/REACTIONS (DYNAMICS).

2. BEHAVIOURAL

According to this theory you may LEARN unsupportive PATTERNS of BEHAVIOUR (such as being passive) to avoid being PUNISHED or to earn PRAISE.

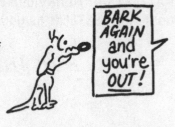

Over time, this type of behaviour leads you to push down your OWN wants and needs in an effort to CONFORM.

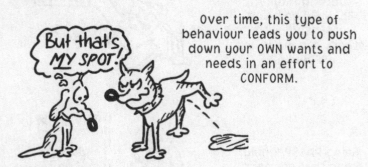

As a result, rather than gaining REWARDS, you will tend to be USED or OVERLOOKED, since you have not learned to set clear BOUNDARIES.

3. PHYSICAL

This theory suggests that you could have been born with a certain brain chemistry or brain structure that could make you more likely to experience DEPRESSION.

Changes in the brain apparently cause dulling of nervous impulses, resulting in depression.

While chemical imbalance may be a CONTRIBUTING factor, it is unlikely to be a SINGLE CAUSE.

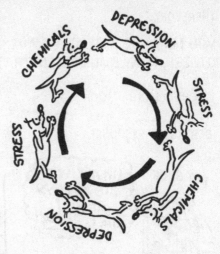

It is still unclear as to which comes FIRST —

CHEMICALS creating MOOD or MOOD creating a CHEMICAL CHANGE!

Regarding GENES, a family history of depression may be HEREDITARY but it could also indicate LEARNED BEHAVIOUR.

At the very WORST, a GENETIC or CHEMICAL imbalance may make you more SUSCEPTIBLE to FEELING DEPRESSED about life than others.

THIS IS AN IMPORTANT POINT, SO LET'S EXPLORE IT:

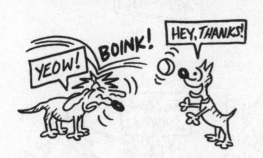

A PREDISPOSITION (chemical or otherwise) to depression may mean that you see life events BOUNCING OFF others, while you experience them as PERSONAL BLOWS!

If you tend to REACT and RESPOND in a depressed way, you will PERCEIVE MORE and MORE 'personal blows' which will ADD to your depression!

41

THEREFORE,

YOU MAY NOT ACTUALLY HAVE MORE HARDSHIP THAN OTHERS, IT WILL JUST SEEM THAT WAY.

Let's take a look:

DEPRESSED RESPONSE

POSITIVE RESPONSE

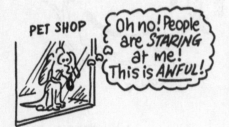

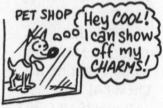

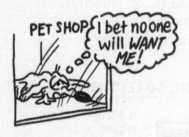

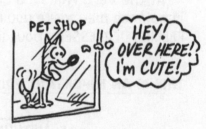

FINAL OUTCOME?

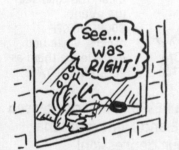

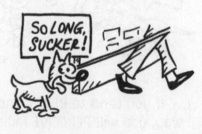

Let's examine how each dog's EXPECTATIONS and PERCEPTIONS of the SAME SITUATION led to a different EXPERIENCE of it for each.

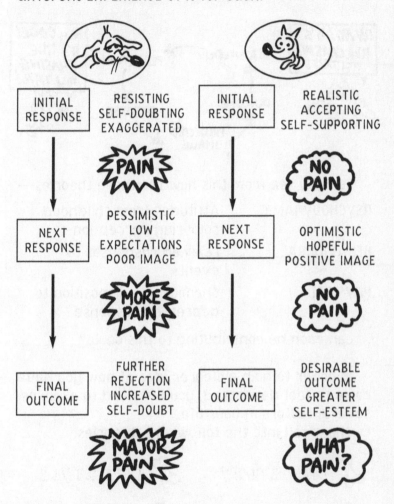

| INITIAL RESPONSE | RESISTING SELF-DOUBTING EXAGGERATED | INITIAL RESPONSE | REALISTIC ACCEPTING SELF-SUPPORTING |

PAIN — **NO PAIN**

| NEXT RESPONSE | PESSIMISTIC LOW EXPECTATIONS POOR IMAGE | NEXT RESPONSE | OPTIMISTIC HOPEFUL POSITIVE IMAGE |

MORE PAIN — **NO PAIN**

| FINAL OUTCOME | FURTHER REJECTION INCREASED SELF-DOUBT | FINAL OUTCOME | DESIRABLE OUTCOME GREATER SELF-ESTEEM |

MAJOR PAIN — **WHAT PAIN?**

If you tend to feel depressed, you will SEE things as DEPRESSING, RESPOND with DEPRESSION & LOOK DEPRESSED, thus inviting DEPRESSING results.

This becomes a VICIOUS CIRCLE.

BUT start out with a DIFFERENT ATTITUDE, and it can become a HAPPY CIRCLE instead! (But we'll get to that later).

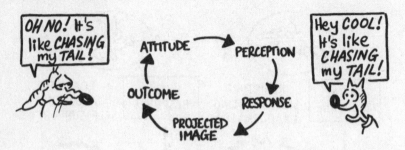

Can you see from this how the three theories —

PSYCHODYNAMIC   Attitudes from childhood
                 colouring perception

BEHAVIOURAL   Learned responses to
                 events

PHYSICAL   Chemical predisposition to
                 depressed response

can each be contributing to this cycle?

In order to gain a clearer idea of how you have come to feel depressed, you will need to examine several factors in your life.

These fall into the following categories:

🦴 LIFE STORY   🦴 LIFE STYLE

🦴 LIFE EVENTS   🦴 PHYSICAL

ANY or ALL of these may have played a part in creating your depression.

LIFE STORY

(A) CHILDHOOD

What sort of childhood did you have?

Did you feel valued, loved, secure and respected?

Did you learn independence and self-worth?

Issues during childhood that may have affected you include:

LACK OF AFFECTION

Your parents may have been too distant, too busy, undemonstrative or of the 'children should be seen and not heard' school.

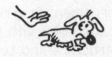

ABUSE

Violent, aggressive or abusive behaviour sends a message to a child that the world is an unsafe, uncaring place.

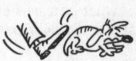

If violence occurs one minute and 'love' the next, the child will be confused and unsure.

SMOTHERING

On the other hand, if you were overly protected and smothered by affection, you may not have learned true independence and may be overly reliant on and affected by others' opinions of you.

HOUSE RULES

An overly strict or
disciplinarian household,
or a household based on
rigid social, religious or
ethnic conventions may
lead you to be 'obedient'
to an extreme or
rebellious as a form of
protest.

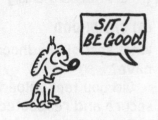

ANYTHING GOES

In contrast to this, an
'anything goes'
environment may not have
provided you with a sense
of structure and security.

While you may not totally fit into these broad
categories, as a child you tend to learn by
example.

What patterns of behaviour and responses to
stress did your parents teach you?

(B) ADULTHOOD

If you were not well equipped in childhood to cope
adequately with the many changes and challenges
in life, adulthood can indeed be a painful journey.

Your self-esteem, if low to start with, can be
further undermined by poor coping skills learned
earlier and not adapted to support you over
time.

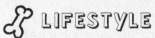 **LIFESTYLE**

In contrast to a challenging life, an UNEVENTFUL
life can contribute to depression, too.

FACTORS HERE INCLUDE:

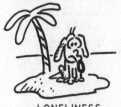

LONELINESS

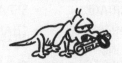

BOREDOM WITH JOB
OR DAILY ROUTINE

LACK OF STIMULATING
INTERESTS OR ACTIVITIES

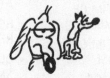

ALIENATION FROM SPOUSE,
PARTNER OR FAMILY

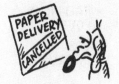

UNEMPLOYMENT

RETIREMENT

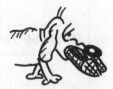

TOO MANY RESPONSIBILITIES
— NOT ENOUGH FUN

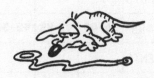

LACK OF FULFILMENT OR
GOALS.

Even normal life events can create accumulated
stress — especially if you don't handle stress well.

In the chart below, tick off the life events you have experienced in the appropriate age bracket, in the colour designated. Red equals high stress.

RED	ORANGE	BLUE
• DEATH OF SOMEONE CLOSE	• ILLNESS OF SOMEONE CLOSE	• BEGINNING/ LEAVING EDUCATION
• MARRIAGE	• SEPARATION	• FALL OUT WITH FRIEND
• DIVORCE	• CHANGE IN JOB OR POSITION	• ILLNESS/ ACCIDENT (LONGER THAN 1 WEEK)
• MOVING OVERSEAS	• CHILD LEAVING HOME	
• MAJOR DEBT BEYOND MEANS	• PERSONAL ACHIEVEMENT	• TRAVEL
• VICTIM OF CRIME	• HOUSE RENOVATION	• DEBT (MEDIUM)
• VICTIM OF ABUSE	• QUITTING SMOKING/ ALCOHOL	• DIETING
• JAIL OR DETENTION		• CHANGE IN SLEEP PATTERN
• MAJOR ILLNESS/ ACCIDENT	• LAW VIOLATION	
• PREGNANCY/ LOSS OF	• MOVING HOUSE	• FALLING IN LOVE
• RETIREMENT	• CHANGE OF SCHOOL	• JOB INTERVIEW
	• DEBT (MORE THAN $10,000)	

YEARS	0–5	6–10	1–15	16–20	21–25	26–30	31–35
EVENTS							
YEARS	36–40	41–45	46–50	51–55	56–60	61–65	66–70
EVENTS							
YEARS	71–75	76–80	81–85	86–90	91–95	95–100	101–105
EVENTS							

IT ALL ADDS UP!!

🦴 PHYSICAL

Changes in your body chemistry can also lead to your feeling depressed.

THESE INCLUDE:

VIRAL INFECTIONS

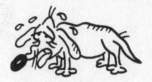

OVERWORK

HORMONAL CHANGES

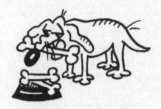

INADEQUATE DIET OR CHANGES IN WEIGHT

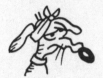

OPERATION OR ILLNESS

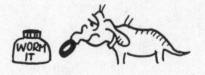

PRESCRIPTION DRUGS

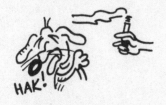

RECREATIONAL DRUGS (AND WITHDRAWAL FROM)

AGEING

If you haven't related to ANY of these, well ...

WELCOME
TO
EARTH!

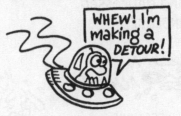

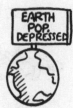

5

BAD DOG!

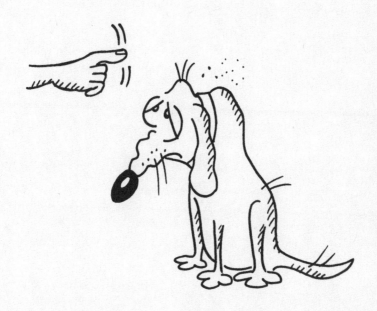

SELF-ESTEEM AND DEPRESSION

EVERYONE on the planet is subject to the stresses of daily life — such as:

MONEY ISSUES

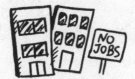

WORK DEMANDS

RELATIONSHIPS

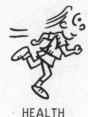

HEALTH

THE NEED
FOR SHELTER

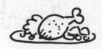

ADEQUATE
FOOD, ETC.

So why is it that some people are able to BREEZE through challenges, while others go under?

The key here centres around an OUTLOOK based on how you feel about YOURSELF.

People will REACT differently to a problem, depending on their attitude to what they feel they DESERVE and their EXPECTATIONS around life.

As we explored in the last chapter, this view is greatly influenced by the messages you were given about your worth when you were a child.

FOR INSTANCE:

If you were CRITICISED, IGNORED, TEASED, BLAMED or ABUSED, you will question your VALUE to the world.

You will not EXPECT much JOY from life.

If, on the other hand, you were PAMPERED, SMOTHERED or OVER-PROTECTED, you may not have learned how to be INDEPENDENT. You may EXPECT a great deal from life, but not get it.

If you were BULLIED or RIDICULED for showing your feelings, you may place great WORTH on appearing TOUGH. You may view life with CYNICISM and ANGER.

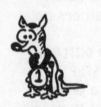

Having to CONFORM, being PUSHED to EXCEL, having to be 'GOOD' may mean that you do not VALUE your own opinions or feelings.
You may see life as OVERWHELMING.

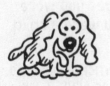

However, if you were NURTURED, SUPPORTED, ENCOURAGED and LOVED you will feel you hold a VALUABLE place in the world.
You will be OPTIMISTIC and REALISTIC about life.

NEGATIVE messages about yourself will tend to create a PATTERN that becomes entrenched as a BELIEF which becomes a REALITY.

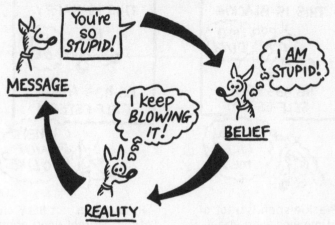

In other words, you will tend to BEHAVE according to your BELIEFS about yourself or life.
POSITIVE messages work in the same way, except the PATTERN reinforces SELF-WORTH!

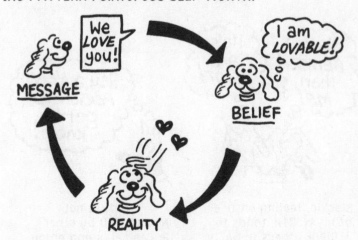

What MESSAGES and BELIEFS in your life have contributed to your current REALITY?

Let's compare the different REALITIES of those with different levels of SELF-WORTH.

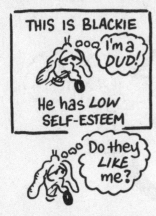

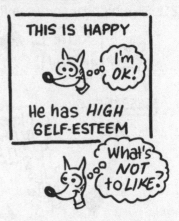

Blackie spends a lot of time worrying about what others think of him. He NEEDS to be liked.

Happy does not RELY on others to feel good about himself. If someone does not engage with him, he knows someone else will.

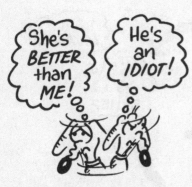

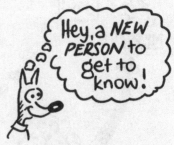

Blackie, feeling unsure of his WORTH, tends to JUDGE others to be BETTER or WORSE.

Happy is not INTIMIDATED by others. He can relax and enjoy them for WHO THEY ARE without COMPARING.

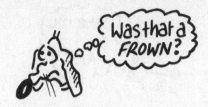

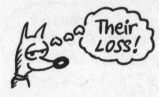

Blackie, needing others' APPROVAL, is ever watchful for signs of REJECTION and cannot RELAX.

Happy is able to DISENGAGE from others' opinions of him. He is thus free to be GENEROUS and EXPANSIVE without fearing being HURT.

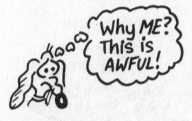

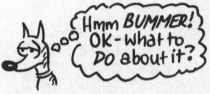

Blackie tends to take life's ups and downs PERSONALLY. He also tends to stay focused on the PAIN, rather than exploring OPTIONS.

Happy sees challenges as part of life, but views them as PROBLEMS needing SOLUTIONS. He moves on QUICKLY, so the pain has less IMPACT.

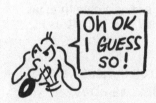

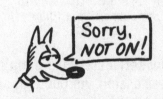

Blackie has trouble setting BOUNDARIES or saying NO. The trouble is, by not setting LIMITS, he feels USED.

Happy only takes on what he WANTS to. Thus he has no need to blame anyone else for his OWN CHOICES.

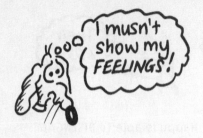

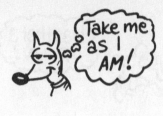

Blackie avoids taking RISKS or stepping out of a certain model of BEHAVIOUR, for fear of being DISAPPROVED of.

Happy believes that ALL parts of his character are what make him UNIQUE. He shows his feelings, accepts his mistakes and is TRUE to himself.

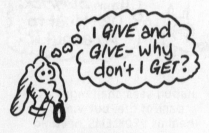

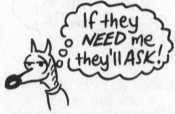

Blackie believes that CARETAKING others will make him more VALUED. Others may LET him, but he will rarely be THANKED for it, because it is a form of CONTROL.

Happy leaves others alone to LEARN and GROW from their own experiences. He respects others' RIGHTS to steer their own lives as THEY see fit, not as HE does.

Low self-esteem is a major factor in your depression. As you can see from the above examples, it will tend to govern the CHOICES you make which affect the DIRECTION your life takes.

A clear understanding of how this operates in your life is necessary for you to make DIFFERENT CHOICES in the future.

What creates SELF-ESTEEM?

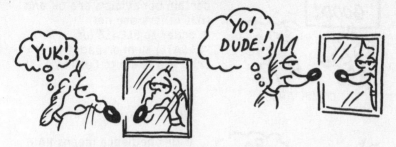

As children, our parents and elders are ALL-POWERFUL figures ... in fact, they are almost GODS. We rely on them for NURTURE, SECURITY and EMOTIONAL care.

They also teach us about LIFE by example.

We seldom QUESTION these teachings because:

(A) We do not have the EXPERIENCE to make comparisons.

(B) We trust in the PROCESS.

(C) We NEED our parents/elders to be RIGHT — for, if not, where does that leave US?

(D) Our very SURVIVAL depends on being LOVED and APPROVED of — i.e. BELONGING.

We will win this LOVE and APPROVAL by various means —

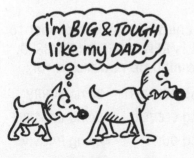

COPYING

A boy sees his father and a girl her mother as the model for being a MAN or a WOMAN. The parent of a child of the opposite gender represents a FIRST LOVE. A child will tend to COPY and DEFEND a parent's behaviour — ANY behaviour!

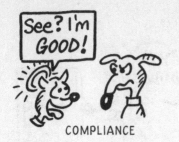

COMPLIANCE

The child soon learns that certain behaviours are OK and that others are not.
In order to PLEASE (or PLACATE) Mum or Dad, the child will learn to COMPLY.

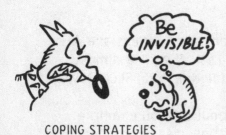

COPING STRATEGIES

If disobedience means PAIN (emotional or physical) and this pain is constant, the child will firstly become PASSIVE (so as not to upset) then SWITCH OFF EMOTIONS (to avoid feeling pain).

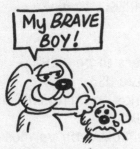

PLAYING THE GAME

Boys don't CRY.
Girls don't LOSE THEIR TEMPER.
If there are RULES that forbid certain EMOTIONS, we may SHUT DOWN on our natural EXPRESSION.

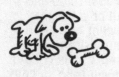

SEEKING REWARD

A child will respond most to what is REWARDED or PRAISED.
We may be rewarded for:

- Being OBEDIENT
- Being CLEVER
- Being QUIET
- Being GOOD
- Being SORRY
- Being INVISIBLE
- Being PASSIVE
- Being TOUGH

Many people with depression will have issues around COMPLIANCE, DEPENDENCY or PASSIVITY.

This PASSIVITY may be disguised under an apparently assertive exterior in some cases, but will be revealed through UNCLEAR BOUNDARIES, DECISIONS BASED ON PLEASING OTHERS, OVER-RELIANCE ON OTHERS' APPROVAL and A NEED TO EXCEL.

If, early on, you learn to be PASSIVE, you may miss out on crucial GROWTH, through RISK TAKING, DECISION MAKING, PROBLEM SOLVING and EXPRESSING OPINIONS and EMOTIONS OPENLY.

'Playing it safe' may mean you end up as a SPECTATOR to life, instead of a KEY PLAYER.

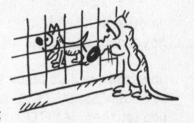

The price we pay for 'ROLLING OVER' may include:

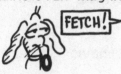

BEING 'USED'

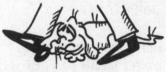

BEING IGNORED

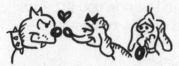

BEING REJECTED

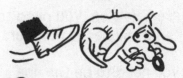

BEING ABUSED

AND ULTIMATELY —

FEELING DEPRESSED!

However, if you think someone 'made' you feel bad or unworthy, think again!

That is only going to be the case if you AGREE with their opinion of you. You can DISAGREE!

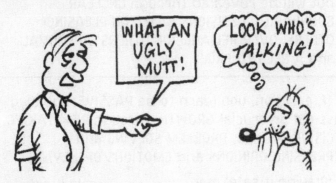

Do others DESERVE to have the privilege of governing your life?

How do their lives look to you? Are they examples of GOODNESS, SUCCESS, KINDNESS? No? Then why do you let them MATTER? Why are their opinions so IMPORTANT?

Don't let someone else's bad behavior justify your being MEAN to YOURSELF!

From now on, YOU need to be the one you RELY ON to fill the needs you wanted others to provide.

You need to be the one you turn TO, not UPON!

If you can't be there for you, who will be?

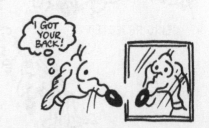

A WORD FOR THE FOLKS

While much of this chapter has centred around childhood issues and, in particular, the type of PARENTING you had, this is not to lay BLAME at the feet of your parents!

There are a few things to keep in mind here.

☆ Your parents were also taught by THEIR parents! That's all they knew.

☆ YOU live in a time when you have the opportunity to grow spiritually BEYOND the limitations of the past.

☆ In other words, you can become BIG enough to accommodate another's SMALLNESS.

☆ While your childhood may have been tough, you have a CHOICE as an ADULT to remain that wounded CHILD, or not.

☆ It is IMPOSSIBLE to be a PERFECT parent.

☆ Your childhood can lead to an important decision in your own life — TO DO BETTER!

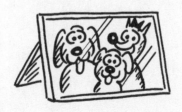

6

'GIVE A DOG A BONE'

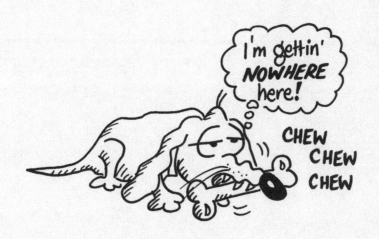

THINKING AND DEPRESSION

Of course, knowing the CAUSE or CAUSES of your depression, or even acknowledging that you have LOW SELF-ESTEEM, is going to remain little more than an ACADEMIC EXERCISE unless you identify how you 'do' your own particular form of depression, and CHANGE that!

IN OTHER WORDS — How do you THINK about having depression, or indeed, LIFE in general?

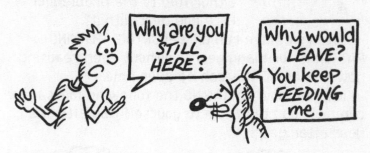

For instance, if you believe that your depression is purely GENETIC (or CHEMICAL) in origin, you might THINK about that in several ways.

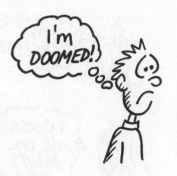

YOU MAY THINK OF YOURSELF AS A VICTIM.

YOU MAY FEEL HELPLESS AND OVERWHELMED THAT THERE IS LITTLE YOU CAN DO ABOUT THIS THING THAT HAS HAPPENED TO YOU.

YOU MAY DREAM ABOUT BEING RESCUED

OR . . .

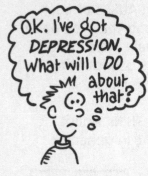

You may decide to ACCEPT that you have a PROBLEM and that you will need to explore ways of living with it. This may, for instance, involve MEDICATION, COUNSELLING, a SUPPORT GROUP OR RETHINKING YOUR LIFE!

Can you see how the two different ways of THINKING can either ADD to the problem or HELP you deal with it?

Often we have run UNSUPPORTIVE THINKING PATTERNS for many years, without even realising how DAMAGING this can be over time.

Imagine how DAMAGING the following messages can be if you tell them to yourself day after day, year after year.

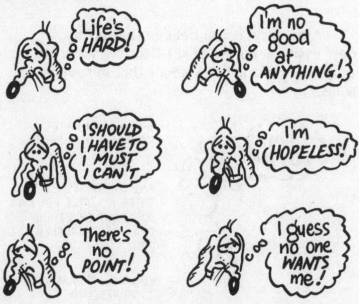

The BLACK DOG is good at TRICKS — especially MENTAL TRICKS that can ADD to your depression (or ANY of life's problems, for that matter). Here are some—

1. AWFULISING

You can feel AWFULLY, TERRIBLY, HORRIBLY depressed or just Depressed. Avoid ADDING to your own discomfort (in ANY situation)!

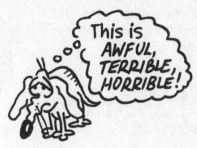

2. RESISTING THE EXPERIENCE

How often do you fight being where you are, doing what you're doing, feeling what you're feeling? How well do you ACCEPT WHAT IS? (And work from there?)

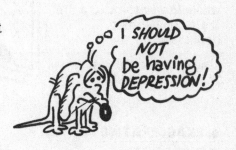

3. WAITING FOR THINGS TO CHANGE

Is your depression going to MAGICALLY DISAPPEAR without you doing anything DIFFERENTLY?

There's a saying: 'If you do what you've always done, you'll get what you've always got.'

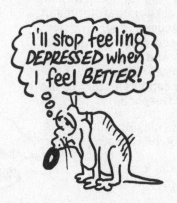

4. BOGGED DOG

There ARE things you can do (this book will show you plenty), but NOTHING will change until you ACT.

Do SOMETHING — ANYTHING — as long as you make a start.

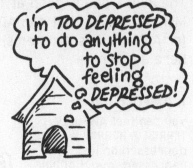

5. CHOICE

You have CHOICE about EVERYTHING.

You can even CHOOSE to let depression take over your whole life or to build a life that's BIGGER than depression.

Stay or move on. Just know that you've CHOSEN.

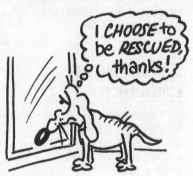

6. EXAGGERATING THE PROBLEM

You may fall into the trap of looking at a lifetime of insecurity, poor decisions, missed opportunities, etc etc, and deciding that it's such a MESS there's no way you can even start to make a difference.

This thinking will OVERWHELM you.

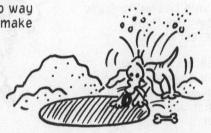

7. UNDERESTIMATING THE TASK

While EXAGGERATING the problem can hold you back, UNDERESTIMATING the effort involved to improve matters, can set you up for DISAPPOINTMENT. What's taken a LIFETIME to build up isn't going to be fixed by one walk around the block!

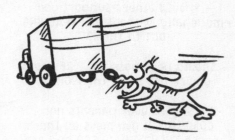

8. COMFORT ZONES

Ironically, over time, your depression is now less threatening than engaging with the WORLD again. Your ESCAPE has become your PRISON.

A tough decision has to be made to step out of your COMFORT ZONE and back into LIFE.

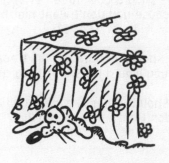

9. SELF-TALK

A dangerous mental trap is the tape that runs constantly in your head and berates you for your MISTAKES, tells you you're a LOSER, or gives you an endless list of RULES about how you, others or the world SHOULD be.

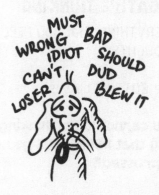

MUST
WRONG BAD
IDIOT SHOULD
CAN'T DUD
LOSER BLEW IT

10. EXPECTATIONS

How REALISTIC are your
EXPECTATIONS of how life should be?

— Should others support you
emotionally, without you REACHING
OUT to THEM?

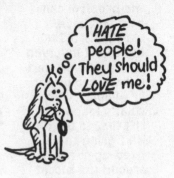

— Should your boss not FIRE you if
you're not doing the WORK?

— Should your parents not
COMPLAIN if you mess up the
house THEY'VE PAID FOR and are
letting you stay in?

— Should your lover STAY just
because you don't want him/her to
LEAVE?

— Should people not DIE because
you would be SAD if they did?

— Should others respect you if you
don't earn or demand RESPECT?

NEGATIVE THINKING

EVERYTHING that you FEEL is governed by your
THOUGHTS.

The BOTTOM LINE is:

**You cannot keep thinking in a negative way — in a
way that DEPRESSES you — and expect not to feel
depressed!!**

Sadness and happiness cannot co-exist.
One cancels out the other.

Whilst actual happiness may seem completely out of reach from where you are at the moment, you can start moving towards at least a feeling of RELIEF by keeping an eye on the nature of your thoughts.

Anytime you're:

- WORRYING
- COMPLAINING
- RESISTING
- RESENTING
- CRITICISING
- BEING PESSIMISTIC
- GETTING STUCK IN THE PAST
- JUDGING
- LAMENTING ...

You're adding to the STOCKPILE of NEGATIVITY.

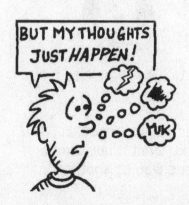

Really? How does THAT work? WHO is doing your THINKING other than YOU?

If YOU'RE not the one in CHARGE of your thoughts, who IS?

If YOU can't get your thoughts working FOR instead of AGAINST you, who CAN?

Your thoughts are really just OPINIONS of things, aren't they? But those opinions carry a lot of weight in determining how you feel.

Put simply:

Tell yourself BAD things and you'll feel BAD!

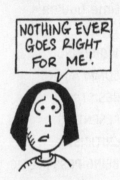

Tell yourself something POSITIVE (that is a real possibility — otherwise you won't believe it) and you'll feel BETTER!

It's really no more mysterious than that!

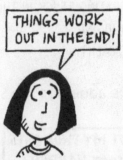

The BIG question is what do you CHOOSE to tell yourself?

What if you changed your opinion from NEGATIVE to HOPEFUL? Or better still, what if you didn't really have an opinion, one way or another?

For example:

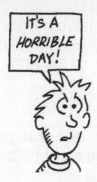

No it isn't. It's just a DAY that you currently THINK is horrible.

Things are just things. Events happen. Until we place an OPINION upon them, they have no particular meaning.

Can you see how much influence you actually have in determining how you experience life?

If you are CHOOSING to stay NEGATIVE, ask yourself how this is SERVING you — because, on some level it is.

Let's take a (hard) look at this—

- INACTION MEANS NO RISK OF FAILURE

- YOU CAN BE TAKEN CARE OF

- YOU GET MORE SYMPATHY, LOVE OR ATTENTION THAN WHEN YOU'RE WELL

- IT'S MORE 'INTERESTING' THAN BEING HAPPY

- YOUR DEPRESSION IS LESS PAINFUL THAN THE CHOICES YOU NEED TO MAKE TO FIX YOUR LIFE (e.g. leaving a relationship)

Assuming that you have bought this book with the intention of getting BETTER, then your thinking needs to CHANGE — no IFs, ANDs or BUTs!

That's the WORK.

It is important to realise that your thoughts are not FACTS — they are just notions.

Compare the difference here:

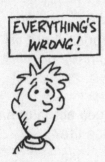 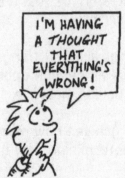

NOTHING is happening TO you!
The THOUGHTS you are putting out there match up with what you EXPECT to happen.
Think of your thoughts as being COMMANDS.

COMMAND   **OUTCOME**

What seems to be happening TO you, is actually coming FROM you!

Change the 'commands' at the outset and you change the OUTCOME!

A WORD ABOUT 'PLAYING DEAD'

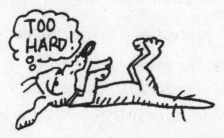

A very common response when you're in a depressed state is to go into retreat from the world. Things 'out there' feel too painful to bear and so you 'disappear' or 'escape' into yourself.

When you do this, it's called NUMBING.

However, in doing so, you are not so much ESCAPING pain from 'out there' as DIGGING DEEPER into your own pain.

Pain — PHYSICAL, EMOTIONAL or even SPIRITUAL — is not there to PUNISH you. Pain shows up to draw your attention to a PROBLEM that needs FIXING.

It simply means that:

- SOMETHING IS OUT OF BALANCE
- SOMETHING NEEDS TO CHANGE.

The problem that needs fixing the most is not the PAIN so much as the REASON you have this pain in the first place.

The trouble is not so much that you have depression in the first place, but that you get stuck on LICKING THE WOUND so that it can never HEAL and only gets WORSE!

The pain of depression is telling you that:

- YOU DON'T LIKE WHERE YOU'RE AT
- YOU DON'T LIKE THE WAY YOU ARE
- YOU HAVEN'T GIVEN YOURSELF ANY CLEAR DIRECTION
- YOU HAVEN'T CREATED A CLEAR PLAN

Isn't that HELPFUL information? Now you know WHY you feel this way!

But instead of addressing these CAUSES of your depression, you tend to become fixated on the depression itself.

And because it feels so PAINFUL, you'll find ways to NUMB that pain, rather than embrace it. These NUMBING responses include:

- DRINKING/DRUGS
- EATING
- GAMBLING
- SHOPPING

- OVERWORKING
- INTERNET
- PROCRASTINATING
- UNHEALTHY RELATIONSHIPS
- TELEVISION

NUMBING might SEEM like COMFORT but it's not —
it's digging DEEPER into a HOLE.

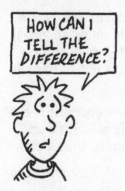

HOW CAN I
TELL THE
DIFFERENCE?

That's EASY — ask yourself:
do you feel GOOD about
yourself when you do it?

Moving beyond numbing means FEELING and of
course, that is the VERY thing you seek to AVOID
through numbing.

The bottom line is: it's PAIN that got you into this,
and that pain can go on FOREVER if you let it. Do
you really WANT that?

Or are you willing to feel the TEMPORARY pain of
lifting off the bandaid so that you can heal?

Feeling (and releasing) PAIN is the way out.

How to do this:

- Be willing to MOVE ON. Enough is ENOUGH.

- Know that you have a right to your feelings. Also know that feelings are actually NATURAL. They come and they go in response to certain stimuli — just like any bodily function.

- NAME the beasts. As your feelings come up, give them a label: 'This is anger', 'This is hurt', 'This is sorrow', etc.

- Now give the feelings a time-zone: 'This is the PAST', or 'This is the FUTURE'. In doing so, you'll see how much of your PRESENT is coloured by what has gone before or what is yet to happen — neither of which you can alter.

- INDULGE the feelings. Don't make yourself feel as though you 'shouldn't' feel this way. Instead, make 'room' to feel this feeling, so that it can move through more easily.

- Stop comparing your pain to anyone else's. They're YOUR feelings — neither BETTER nor WORSE than anyone else's.

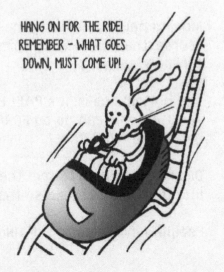

HANG ON FOR THE RIDE! REMEMBER — WHAT GOES DOWN, MUST COME UP!

- If all else fails, ride out the cycle till it PASSES. It DOES pass — every time!

7

The Training Begins

TOP DOG

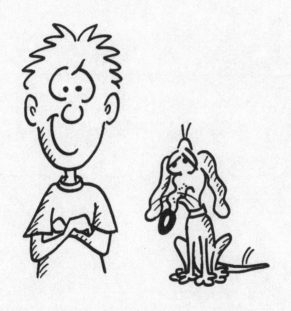

REASSESSING DEPRESSION

By now, hopefully, you will have a clearer picture of how you came to be depressed and how the BLACK DOG's tricky thinking ADDS to the problem.

Now you need to ASSESS how you can APPROACH this problem in a new way, in order to HANDLE it better.

What you have on your hands is a BLACK DOG that needs DISCIPLINE, DIRECTION and TRAINING IN NEW SKILLS.

You want your BLACK DOG to FOLLOW YOUR LEAD — not pull you off track!

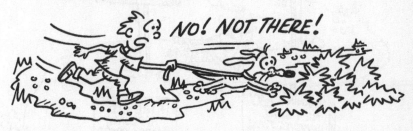

NO! NOT THERE!

And the only way to do this is to become TOP DOG.

You need to ask yourself —

Who's in CHARGE?

In other words —

> Do I rule my life or does
> my depression?
> How much of my THINKING
> centres around the PROBLEM
> instead of a SOLUTION?
> Have I allowed my
> depression to TAKE OVER?

If Blackie is in charge, then YOU will need to STEER him back on course.

This will involve adopting a more SUPPORTIVE view of the PROBLEM itself, to keep you on track.

SUCH AS ...

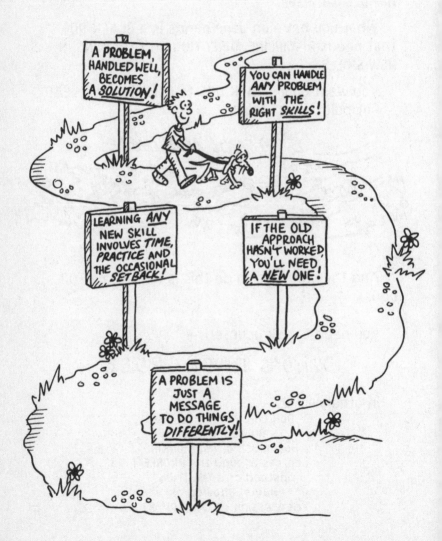

Recovery involves 4 main decisions —

🦴 To WANT to get WELL

🦴 To risk DISCOMFORT to get well

🦴 To be prepared to make CHANGES

🦴 To BEGIN, and then to CONTINUE.

These decisions
may appear obvious,
but you are likely to
stall on any one of
them, because they
can involve revealing
and acknowledging
that there are parts of yourself that are not
always noble, and other parts where you have
buried old pain.

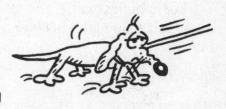

To make a commitment to recovery, you will
need to apply a lot of SELF-HONESTY and a
willingness to MOVE PAST that which has held you
back thus far.

At this point, it would be good to acknowledge:

Until I face my own Shadow,
I will see it in my life.

In other words, you're going to keep tripping
up on what you're trying to AVOID.

In POSITIVE terms, this whole process could be seen as simply a means of building up your EMOTIONAL MUSCLE, so that your weak spots no longer cause you injury!

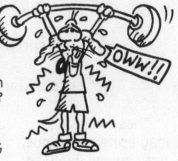

SELF-HONESTY is the greatest EMOTIONAL MUSCLE BUILDER there is. After all, if you keep TRIPPING YOURSELF UP, how can any OUTSIDE factor be of help?

Being honest with yourself may mean OWNING UP TO:

- SELF-PITY

- INACTIVITY

- WANTING TO BE RESCUED

- BLAMING OTHERS/LIFE FOR YOUR SITUATION

- WANTING TO BE LOOKED AFTER

- BEING ABLE TO CONTROL OTHERS.

Whew!

SELF-HONESTY is not easy, but it results in great FREEDOM. By identifying your TRICKS and removing them, you learn to VALUE and TRUST your INTEGRITY.

So let's look at the four MAIN DECISIONS from a very HONEST point of view.

 ### WANTING TO GET WELL

Often we say we want to do something when what we REALLY want is something to be done FOR us or for it to just HAPPEN. Recovery requires WORK. Are you READY GO FOR IT!

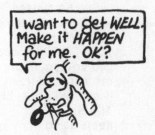

 ### RISKING DISCOMFORT

Self honesty can be UNCOMFORTABLE. Getting up and doing SOMETHING, ANYTHING, can be UNCOMFORTABLE. Choosing not to shut down or hide out can be UNCOMFORTABLE. Reaching out, facing old pain, showing your feelings can all be UNCOMFORTABLE. But your DEPRESSION will only last as long as you AVOID moving on, and through, these things.

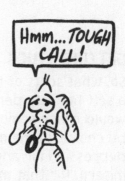

MAKING CHANGES

If it's NOT WORKING, find something that DOES.
If it's OVER, move on.
If it no longer SERVES you, LET IT GO.
How can you expect a DIFFERENT OUTCOME if you repeat the same MISTAKES?

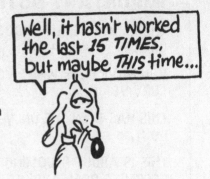

Well, it hasn't worked the last *15 TIMES*, but maybe *THIS* time...

TO BEGIN AND TO CONTINUE

Just reading this book will not produce your RECOVERY.
BEGIN. No matter what, no matter how, DO SOMETHING.
Then CONTINUE what you've begun. Once off won't do it.
If you fall over, BEGIN AGAIN.
Keep going.
You CAN do it. In TIME.

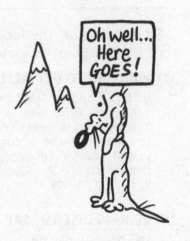

Oh well... Here GOES!

GETTING STUCK

So, what sorts of things (from a self-honesty perspective) would cause someone to stay, by choice, in the misery of depression (or any other misery, for that matter)?

A TRUE COMMITMENT to being well involves a decision to NOT REMAIN where you are, to set a CLEAR GOAL about where you want to be and to DO WHATEVER IS REQUIRED to get there.

Are you COMMITTED? GREAT!

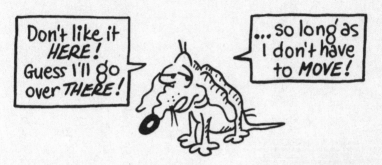

NOW IT'S TIME TO GET TO WORK!

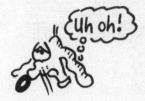

8

ROLLING IN IT

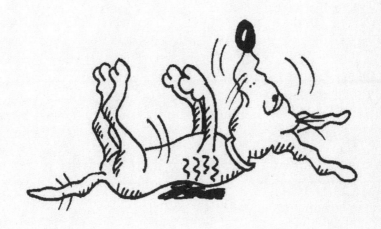

THE TRAP OF SELF-PITY
(WARNING — TOUGH LOVE CHAPTER!)

You've probably been doing a lot of THIS, haven't you?

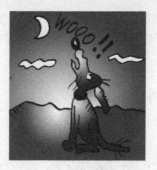

There you are, crying in the night about the UNFAIRNESS of the world and your lot.

In fact, you couldn't really have depression without doing this, so we need to take a good look at what you're spending your TIME and ENERGY on.

If you're depressed, it's pretty certain that you spend a lot of time THINKING about:

THE PAST

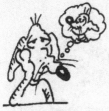

YOUR LOSSES

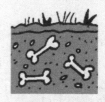

COMPARISON TO OTHERS

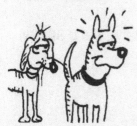

REGRETS

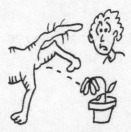

You also probably spend a great deal of time thinking or talking about how BAD you think things are with:

THE STATE OF THE WORLD

PEOPLE

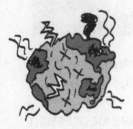

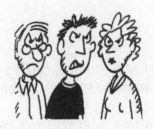

and your SITUATION.

You're also most likely sitting in the DARK, watching a lot of DARK MOVIES and reading DARK NOVELS or searching out DARK THINGS on the internet mainly because doing so confirms and justifies your current bleak outlook.

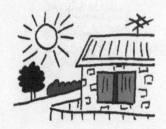

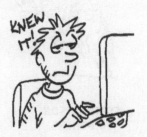

And above all, you're feeling very, very SORRY for yourself.

Whilst you may have EVERY REASON in the world to feel this way, ROLLING in your misery is NOT going to help you feel LESS DEPRESSED, is it?

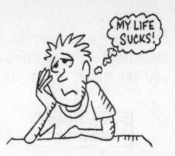

Whilst terrible events or losses may have led you to become depressed, if you want to MOVE ON, it is important to look at — and let go of — the ways you are KEEPING yourself depressed.

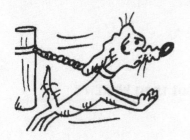

Firstly, you need to lose the idea that you are chained to depression by OUTSIDE FACTORS.

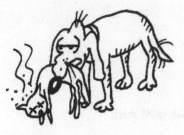

A great deal of how you feel in the moment lies in what you are DRAGGING INTO it, usually from the PAST.

'If only' is the mantra of the depressed, but it's a road to nowhere. You are where you are; it is the way it is.

'If only' means lamenting that which hasn't happened!

Acceptance of your situation and your history is an important step forward. You are here because you are here; that's just the way it is.

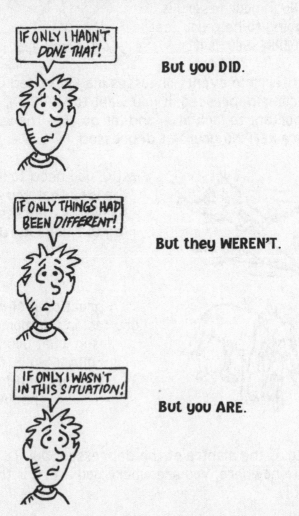

But you DID.

But they WEREN'T.

But you ARE.

When you can accept that you have arrived at this place by the CHOICES you have made (even if you thought you had no choice — you chose to

RESPOND in a certain way), you can use the experience to make BETTER choices from here on.

Dragging the past around is like setting off for a week's trek and lugging provisions for twenty years with you!

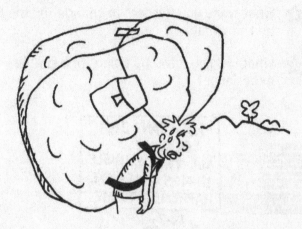

You can only bear 24 hours' worth of experiences at a time. Anything more than that will bog you down.

That means leaving behind not only the business of the PAST but unhelpful projections into the FUTURE as well.

Take one day at a time, and at the end of each day do a review, consciously let it go and start fresh tomorrow.

YOU CANNOT CHANGE THE PAST. IT'S DONE; BUT YOU CAN CHANGE THE IMPACT THAT THE PAST HAS ON YOU BY 'REFRAMING' IT.

REFRAMING THE PAST:

☆ Write down a list of the toughest situations in your life that you thought you would never survive. Now write down what happened next. Was it for the better?

☆ What were you 'forced' to change for the better by the situation?

☆ What did you learn by going through the experience?

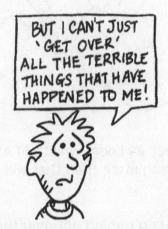

BUT I CAN'T JUST 'GET OVER' ALL THE TERRIBLE THINGS THAT HAVE HAPPENED TO ME!

Again, you may feel you have EVERY REASON in the world to feel sorry for yourself and many people might agree with you, but getting snagged on SELF-PITY is like chasing your tail — it does nothing to CHANGE the situation or the outcome.

There is not one TRULY EVOLVED person on the planet who has not been tested to their limit, often through great LOSS and PAIN. You don't get to be evolved by living a 'safe' life.

The difference is that these people used their experiences to EXPAND, rather than as an excuse for their LIMITATIONS.

You may be stuck, but nothing 'out there' or 'back then' is KEEPING you stuck except your ATTACHMENT to these things.

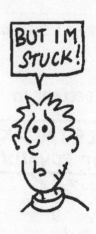

Ask yourself: How long do I intend fo STAY stuck?

Another 5 years? 20 years? For the REST OF MY LIFE?

Do you REALLY want that? Do you want to condemn yourself to endless SUFFERING because of something that happened 10, 20, 30 years ago?

Let go of the 'story'. Stop letting it DEFINE you. Be the person who became a BETTER person BECAUSE of what happened!

Facing down self-pity can be TOUGH but LIBERATING. The temptation to find 'sickly comfort' from self-pity is persuasive but it is a poisonous trap.

Did your childhood or the incident that led to your depression cause your marriage to fail, for you to lose your job, to go broke or whatever has happened?

Indirectly, perhaps, because you learned a way of being that undermined you; but you are not back there anymore, unless you keep dragging it with you into every new situation. The CHOICES you have made have been your OWN.

If your history has led you to make a MESS, you need to:

OWN IT!

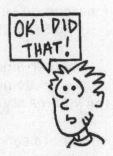

DECLARE IT!

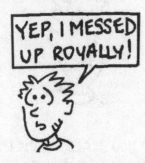

FORGIVE YOURSELF FOR IT!

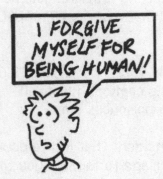

FIX IT!

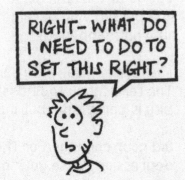

A line by Werner Erhardt (founder of *est*, later Landmark Forum — a radical self-improvement course from the 1970s) is: *Giving sympathy to the self-pitying is like giving a drink to an alcoholic.*

Harsh, but true.

The trouble with self-pity is that it's addictive and if you get 'rewarded' by sympathy, you'll keep coming back for more — which means you need to keep holding on to the problem.

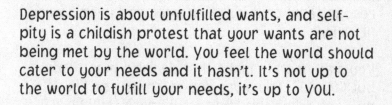

Depression is about unfulfilled wants, and self-pity is a childish protest that your wants are not being met by the world. You feel the world should cater to your needs and it hasn't. It's not up to the world to fulfill your needs, it's up to YOU.

Another quote, from *The Blazing World*, a novel by Siri Hustvedt:

> *Sadness, Anton, I said, is because of self-grasping. We are all looking for things to satisfy this sense of want that we feel will satisfy our needs. We all know that the want will appear and the next and so on, but when we put it on the shelf, we can move beyond it.*

What this is saying is that your wants will never be fully satisfied, either. It is what keeps us searching, inventing, creating. It's human nature to desire more.

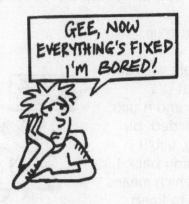

Don't think yourself WRONG for indulging in self-pity now and then (we all do it), but learn to recognise when it is taking over and keeping you HELPLESS.

You may need to make that decision many times, but MAKE IT. The more you catch yourself in self-pity and make this choice, the more EMPOWERED you will feel and the more likely you will be to take positive action.

Basically, depression without self-pity cannot exist.

Stepping out of that trap is your key to FREEDOM.

9

DOG BITES

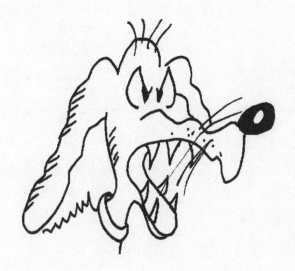

THE ROLE OF ANGER
IN DEPRESSION

WHO or WHAT are you really ANGRY with?

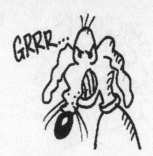

Because that's what is at the heart of the PROBLEM, isn't it? You feel ANGRY about something you feel you have been DEPRIVED of or a situation you think you can't FIX.

You might feel angry towards:

GOD OR FATE

PEOPLE WHO HAVE HURT YOU

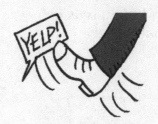

THE 'UNFAIRNESS' OF A SITUATION

OR

THOSE WHO HAVE 'ABANDONED' YOU.

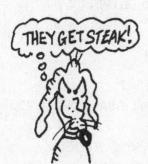

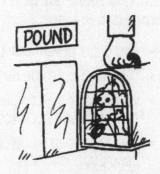

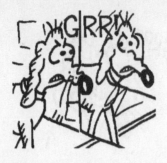

But most likely, the
one you are most
angry with is
YOURSELF.

Sigmund Freud referred to depression as anger
turned inward and we need to spend a little time
exploring the role of ANGER in relation to your
DEPRESSION.

When you become angry with yourself, an INNER
BULLY emerges.

This bully tells you
that you are:

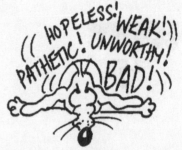

This inner anger is often anger towards OTHERS
that you have not been able to OUTWARDLY
express because:

- YOU WERE DEPENDENT ON THEM

- THEY HAD CONTROL OVER YOU

- YOU FEARED THAT YOU WOULD BE ABANDONED IF YOU
  SHOWED YOUR FEELINGS

- YOU FEARED BEING REJECTED IF YOU WEREN'T
  COMPLIANT OR NICE.

SELF HATE can be described as 'taking revenge on yourself for the faults of others.'

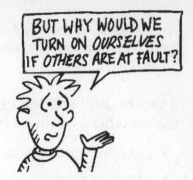

BUT WHY WOULD WE TURN ON *OURSELVES* IF *OTHERS ARE AT FAULT?*

The origins of this are usually to be found in our formative years.

We figure that it is best to blame ourselves first, rather than try to tackle STRONG, POWERFUL or INTIMIDATING people.

THEY'RE SCARY!

We may also be afraid to see FAULT in those who are meant to love and support us (our 'caretakers') because we fear our very SURVIVAL is at risk.

IT CAN'T BE *THEM SO IT* MUST BE ME!

This is often driven by a desperate need to be LOVED by others, to fill the HOLE in ourselves. If others let us down in this regard, we conclude that it must be because we are WRONG, BAD or UNLOVABLE in some way and that WE are the CAUSE of the problem.

The thing is, no matter how unkind others may have been to you, this anger towards yourself is downright CRUEL.

It causes you to do the very things that you feared others would do to you, such as:

- ABANDONMENT
- HARSH JUDGEMENT
- SELF SABOTAGE
- SELF HARM
- LONELINESS

ANGER in itself is not necessarily a BAD thing. Anger can MOTIVATE you, help you to STAND UP for what you believe and can help you to ASSERT in a healthy way by setting clear BOUNDARIES.

You can actually use anger to help with your SELF ANGER! If you recognise that you are carrying anger that you really feel towards those who have hurt you, you need to GET IT OUT. It has turned inwards because you have not EXPRESSED it to those you are really angry with.

Go ahead:

PUNCH A PILLOW   **YELL UNDERWATER**

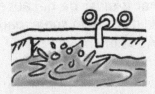

SCREAM IN YOUR CAR

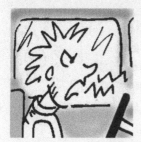

BASH SOMETHING INANIMATE

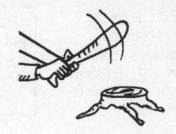

WRITE A LETTER
(BUT DON'T SEND IT!)

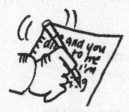

SPEAK IT OUT
(TALK TO A CHAIR AS A STAND-IN
FOR THE OTHER PERSON)

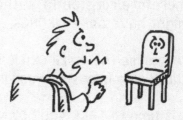

OK, now you've got that out, it's time to recognise that beating yourself up is just like CHASING YOUR TAIL.

No matter what you do, you can't get OTHERS to fix this for you. They may never APOLOGISE, be as LOVING as you want them to be or even believe that they've done anything WRONG!

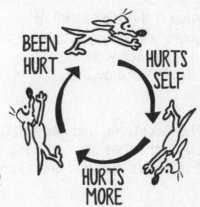

BEEN HURT

HURTS SELF

HURTS MORE

Where does that leave you?

YOU need to rescue you because THEY WON'T. It's simply not their job to do so.

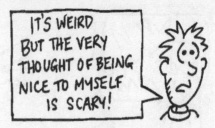

IT'S WEIRD BUT THE VERY THOUGHT OF BEING NICE TO MYSELF IS SCARY!

That is because you have become used to feeling that you have to monitor yourself for any 'slip-ups' that might get others offside. You are therefore constantly on the lookout for what you might have done WRONG.

Recognise the INNER CRITIC for what it is — a CRUEL BULLY who is pushing you into SUFFERING.

It is time to TAKE YOUR OWN SIDE and defend yourself against this constant unkind attack.

HOW DO I DO THAT?

What if a good FRIEND of yours was being attacked in this way? Would you allow this to go on?

The first thing you need to do is to actually HEAR this stuff that you're telling yourself. Say out loud the things that you are saying INSIDE.

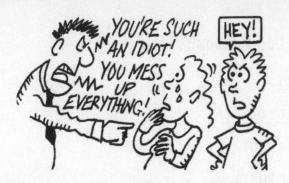

SHOCKING, isn't it? No wonder you feel BAD!

Now you can use your ANGER to CHALLENGE the ideas that this bully is beating you with.

Think about it:

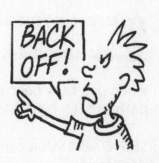

Are you REALLY any worse than most other people? Do you REALLY deserve to SUFFER so much?

Have you just made some MISTAKES instead of committing terrible 'crimes'?

Didn't you do the best you could with what you knew?

Aren't you just a NORMAL, FLAWED HUMAN BEING?

Do you or your friend DESERVE to be PUNISHED in this way?

Use your anger now to fight FOR YOU!

Some DOs AND DON'Ts though:

Do NOT

☆ BE EXPLOSIVE

☆ ACT OUT

☆ BE BITTER.

DO

☆ STAND UP FOR YOURSELF

☆ BELIEVE IN YOUR WORTH

☆ CHALLENGE OTHERS' NEGATIVE JUDGMENTS OF YOU.

When you take your own side, you start down the path of SELF COMPASSION.

SELF COMPASSION can significantly reduce depression.

SELF COMPASSION involves:

☆ SELF-KINDNESS

☆ MINDFULNESS

☆ AN AWARENESS OF COMMON HUMANITY.

Give yourself a BREAK. You did the best you could.

10

DOG EAT DOG

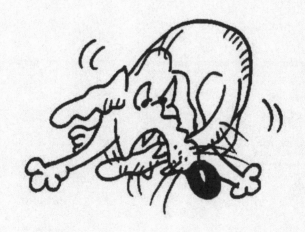

SELF-HARM

Some people resort to SELF-HARM as a way of coping with emotional and psychological pain.

As counter-intuitive as it may seem to an onlooker, those who self-harm do so because the practice brings them RELIEF.

SELF-HARMING may include:

⭐ CUTTING OR SCRATCHING THE SKIN

⭐ BURNING OR SCALDING

⭐ HITTING YOURSELF

⭐ BANGING HEAD AGAINST WALL

⭐ PUNCHING THINGS

⭐ THROWING SELF AGAINST HARD OBJECTS

⭐ STICKING SHARP OBJECTS INTO SKIN

⭐ PREVENTING WOUNDS FROM HEALING

⭐ SWALLOWING DANGEROUS SUBSTANCES/OBJECTS.

However, there are less extreme or obvious forms of self-harm, including:

⭐ RECKLESS DRIVING

⭐ BINGE-DRINKING

⭐ HEAVY DRUG USE

⭐ RISKY BEHAVIOR

⭐ PROMISCUITY.

Self-harm is actually another form of NUMBING —
an attempt to escape EMOTIONAL pain through
PHYSICAL pain. It can act as:

⭐ A DISTRACTION

⭐ A WAY TO OUTWARDLY EXPRESS FEELINGS

⭐ A WAY TO DEAL WITH EARLIER ABUSE OR TRAUMA

⭐ A RESPONSE TO NEGATIVE FEELINGS ABOUT
YOURSELF OR YOUR BODY.

Although it may seem to help in the moment, any
feeling of relief is short-lived and so the person
will self-harm again.

It's a vicious cycle and one that most self-harmers
are not proud of and will often keep secret.

SIGNS OF SELF-HARM

⭐ WEARING CLOTHING THAT COVERS THE WOUNDS
(EVEN IN VERY WARM WEATHER)

⭐ UNEXPLAINED INJURIES

⭐ FREQUENT 'ACCIDENTS', OR
'CLUMSINESS'

⭐ BLOOD STAINS

⭐ CARRYING OR STORING
SHARP OBJECTS

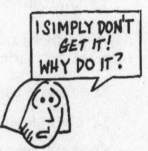

⭐ DISAPPEARING INTO THE BATHROOM OR BEDROOM
FOR LONG PERIODS

⭐ IRRITABILITY AND DEFENSIVENESS

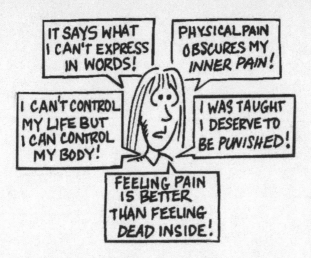

Because self-harm often arises from deep TRAUMA, it is wise to seek professional help to work through the painful feelings you are trying to mask.

Clearly, self-harm is not a helpful option! There are other ways to relieve stress and release strong emotions:

☆ USE WRITING, DRAWING OR SCULPTURE TO EXPRESS YOUR FEELINGS

☆ GET STRENUOUSLY PHYSICAL — RUN, STOMP OR HIT A PUNCHING BAG

☆ YELL OR SCREAM INTO A PILLOW.

Instead of cutting, try:

☆ FLICKING A RUBBER BAND

☆ RUBBING ICE ON YOUR SKIN

☆ USE A RED PEN TO SIMULATE A WOUND.

FETCH!

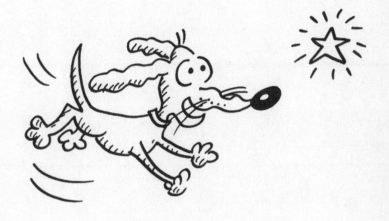

GOING FOR RECOVERY

TRAINING your BLACK DOG involves finding WORKABLE SOLUTIONS to enable you to handle him better, so that he no longer keeps you STUCK.

Each of the KEY AREAS that we have looked at in previous chapters can be approached in a new way, to produce a DIFFERENT ATTITUDE leading to a BETTER OUTCOME.

These KEY AREAS include:

☆ THE PROBLEM ITSELF

☆ THINKING AND DEPRESSION

☆ CHILDHOOD ISSUES

☆ SELF-ESTEEM

☆ DEALING WITH LIFE

☆ PHYSICAL FACTORS.

Remember our comparison between BLACKIE and HAPPY?

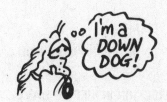 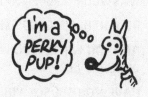

The aim here is to close the gap in your current PERCEPTION of things and move you more in the direction of Happy's view of the world.

THE PROBLEM ITSELF

You've probably been viewing your depression as if it has just 'happened' to you by CHANCE, or through CIRCUMSTANCES beyond your CONTROL.

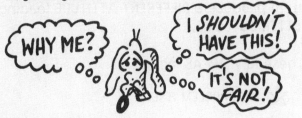

Happy's view

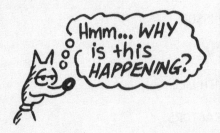

Happy is taking RESPONSIBILITY for the PROBLEM being in his life. He looks for the REASONS why he has this problem.

Take a look at your life, given all the information you have gained so far. Ask yourself ...

- WAS YOUR CHILDHOOD PERFECT?

- DO YOU HAVE GOOD SELF-ESTEEM?

- ARE YOU WHERE YOU WANT TO BE, WITH WHOM YOU WANT TO BE?

- HAVE YOU CHOSEN YOUR DIRECTION IN LIFE OR HAVE OTHERS?

- DO YOU GET BACK AS MUCH AS YOU GIVE?

- IS YOUR LIFESTYLE HEALTHY AND BALANCED?

- ARE YOU ABLE TO FREELY EXPRESS FEELINGS?

- ARE YOU ABLE TO SAY 'NO'?
- DO YOU FEEL FREE OF PAST HURTS?
- DO YOU LOOK AFTER YOURSELF AS WELL AS YOU DO OTHERS?

If you answered 'No' to even HALF of these questions, wouldn't you say that it is NOT SURPRISING that you feel DEPRESSED?

So instead of taking the view of 'WHY ME?' you could take the view of ...

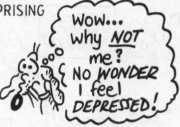

Solutions?

☆ Your depression has simply HIGHLIGHTED existing VULNERABILITIES.
Now they're IDENTIFIED, you can STRENGTHEN them.

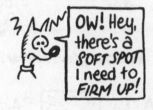

☆ Right now, you are having an EXPERIENCE called depression. If you look at the thinking above, you may realise WHY you are having this experience.
ATTEND to what this experience is asking you to!

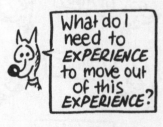

☆ Stop FIGHTING where you are. Work on it till you're SOMEWHERE ELSE!

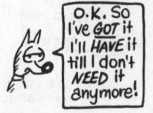

Do you TELL YOURSELF ...

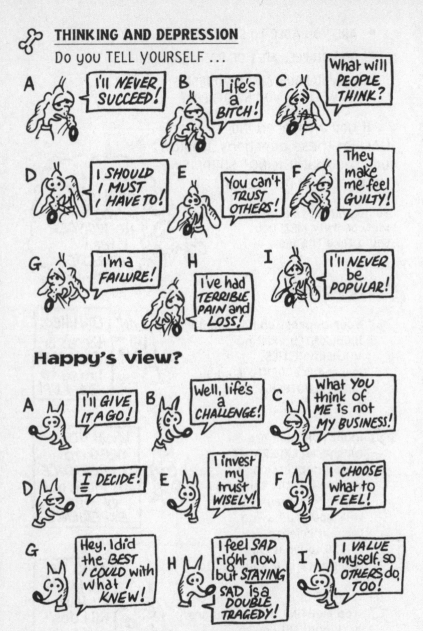

Happy's view?

Which messages would best SUPPORT you?
Which attitude is more ATTRACTIVE?

If you really want to be LESS DEPRESSED, then beware of the self-talk that DEPRESSES you!
Ask yourself this:

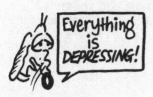

- If I want to feel better, can I AFFORD to keep talking to myself in a NEGATIVE WAY?

- Is what I tell myself SUPPORTING or UNDERMINING me?

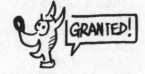

- Would I tell my BEST FRIEND the same messages?

CHOOSE your thoughts with GREAT CARE.
Thoughts are the FUEL for your emotions. Fill up with DOWNERS and you'll be running on MISERY!

Solutions?

☆ Monitor yourself closely for a while. Be aware of what messages you keep running.

☆ If you don't like the station, SWITCH CHANNELS. Challenge the thought. Explore other options.

☆ Omit, as much as possible, all the SHOULDS, MUSTS and HAVE TOs.
   Try 'COULD', 'MIGHT' or 'IF I CHOOSE' instead.

CHILDHOOD ISSUES

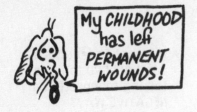

You may, indeed, have had a TERRIBLE and TRAUMATIC childhood that still affects you.

Happy's view

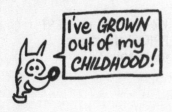

Happy is saying two things here —
(a) That he has 'GROWN OUT OF' i.e. LEFT BEHIND — his childhood.
(b) He has 'GROWN' BECAUSE OF his childhood — meaning that his early trials served as a catalyst to be BIGGER and BETTER than what he began with.

Solutions?

☆ Refuse to stay LOCKED IN to HISTORY. You cannot change the PAST, but you can change how you view it in the present.

☆ Choose not to engage with others and the world through WOUNDS.

☆ Recognise that, as an ADULT, you can choose to remain a CHILD or not.

☆ LEARN from your past. Do it DIFFERENTLY. Decide to (e.g.) give more LOVE, be more PATIENT, have more SUCCESS than you got before.

PUTDOWNS FROM THE PAST

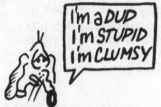

If part of your self-talk includes PUTDOWNS like these — ask yourself where and from whom these ideas of yourself began.

Happy's view:

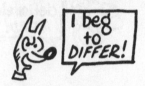

Happy has recognised that these putdowns will only cause pain if he BELIEVES them!

Solutions?

☆ Stop BELIEVING someone ELSE'S opinion of you!

☆ Stop making these putdowns TRUE!

☆ Learn to say 'That's THEIR stuff' instead of automatically taking on criticism.

FORGIVING THE PAST

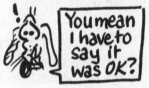

NO! FORGIVENESS is about FREEING YOURSELF from the effects of the past.

FORGIVENESS IS —

☆ RELEASING THE PAST

☆ EMOTIONAL CLOSURE

☆ NO LONGER ATTACHING TO OLD PAIN

☆ DISENGAGING FROM ORIGINAL HURT

☆ ACCEPTING WHAT <u>WAS</u>, CAN'T BE CHANGED, BUT WHAT <u>IS</u> CAN

Happy's view:

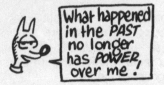

Happy has recognised that emotions like SHAME, GUILT, ANGER or FEAR that he may carry from the past keep HIM a VICTIM of the past.

If you think about it, it's pretty strange to torture YOURSELF more than those who originally caused you pain!

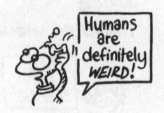

Solutions?

☆ Right here, right now, REFUSE to remain a VICTIM of the past.

Here is your statement of FREEDOM

> X (someone's name), I hereby release you from MY anger, MY pain, MY fear and MY guilt. Go in peace and so will I.

- Do this little ritual, by yourself, for yourself.

RELEASING THE PAST

- Face one end of a room and imagine before you all of the sad, hurtful, painful things of the past piled on top of one another. Pile it all up, gather it all together in one big heap.

- Look at that pile of junk and let yourself FEEL all the emotions that come up. Let them go, release them. Grieve, weep.

- Now turn and face the other end of the room. This is your future, free of baggage. Embrace it.

🦴 <u>SELF-ESTEEM</u>

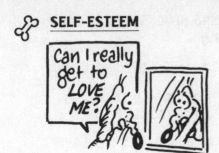

Self-esteem means you CARE ENOUGH for yourself that you SUPPORT yourself in all your DECISIONS, CHOICES, RESPONSES and REACTIONS.

While this may be simple in PRINCIPLE, getting there can be hard, especially if you've had a lot of blows to your self-worth.

Happy's view:

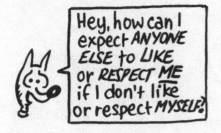

Happy has figured out that what he GIVES OUT is what he will GET BACK.

Let's look at a few of these —

⭐ If you give out HELPLESSNESS, you're going to be treated like a CHILD.

⭐ If you give out GUILT, you'll get back SHAME.

⭐ If you give out RESENTMENT, how are you going to get back LOVE?

⭐ If you give out MISERY, are you going to uplift others? Are they going to ENJOY being with you?

The biggest STUMBLING BLOCKS to self-esteem come from the following —

⭐ OVEREMPHASIS ON OTHERS' OPINIONS OF YOU

⭐ ALLOWING OTHERS OR CIRCUMSTANCES TO DICTATE THE DIRECTION YOUR LIFE TAKES

⭐ NOT SETTING CLEAR BOUNDARIES (i.e. SAYING 'YES' WHEN YOU MEAN 'NO'

⭐ FEELING THAT THIS IS ALL YOU DESERVE AND NOT SEEKING MORE

⭐ BAD PRESS ON YOURSELF (i.e. NEGATIVE SELF-TALK, etc.)

Let's examine these —

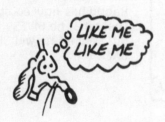

1. OTHERS' OPINIONS

Living your life to please others can NEVER work, simply because it's IMPOSSIBLE to please everybody all of the time.

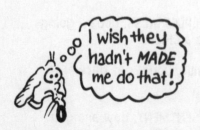

2. LIFE DIRECTION

No one and nothing can MAKE you do something unless you have AGREED to it on some level.

For example, if you were LIED to, ask yourself 'What do I give out that says it's OK to do that to me?'

3. BOUNDARIES

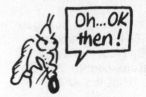

Agreeing to something you don't want is NOT LOVING.
If you are doing it because you WANT approval or DON'T WANT disapproval, then it is not a gift.
A gift has no price tag.

4. ALL I DESERVE

If you place LIMITATIONS on your life, don't be surprised if your life is LIMITED!

5. BAD PRESS

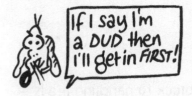

You're going to LIVE OUT what you TELL YOURSELF.

IMPORTANT THOUGHT —
'We teach others how to treat us.'

Solutions?

☆ See others' approval as a BONUS, not a NECESSITY.

☆ Take full responsibility for your OWN life. Live it how YOU want to, not how OTHERS do.

☆ Practise saying 'NO'. Risk rejection.
Be clear about what you want.

☆ Examine your beliefs about what your RIGHTS, CAPABILITIES and EXPECTATIONS are.
Could they be modified?

☆ Avoid 'I AM' statements that limit you.

☆ Be your own fan club!

🦴 DEALING WITH LIFE

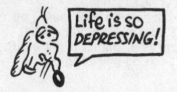

Life is life. It's how you SEE it that makes it DIFFICULT or EASY. Lately, you've DECIDED that it's HARD.

Happy's view:

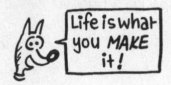

We looked at this point in some detail in Chapter 2.

The biggest stumbling block to handling life is —

WE EXPECT THINGS TO BE PERMANENT!

It's SO OBVIOUS, but most of us still don't GET IT!

Nothing can cause greater misery than trying to fight CHANGE.

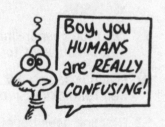

The only thing PERMANENT in life is CHANGE!

When we resist CHANGE, we expect that:

- Things should never BREAK or WEAR OUT

- MONEY should always BE THERE

- People's FEELINGS should never change.

- Your JOB should always be there when you WANT

- People should never LEAVE US, GET SICK or DIE

- We should not AGE, etc.

Can you see how holding on to these expectations leads to DISAPPOINTMENT, FRUSTRATION, RESENTMENT and SADNESS if things turn out DIFFERENTLY?

Solutions?

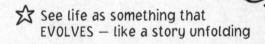

⭐ See life as something that EVOLVES — like a story unfolding

⭐ Expect CHANGE and learn to roll with it

⭐ Reduce your EXPECTATIONS about how things SHOULD be

⭐ One door closes, another opens. Explore other possibilities.

PHYSICAL FACTORS

Certain PHYSICAL FACTORS can contribute to feelings of depression, or can mimic depression.

It is a good idea to get a PHYSICAL CHECK-UP to discount any physical imbalance.

FACTORS MAY INCLUDE:

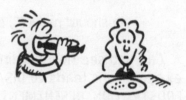

HORMONAL CHANGES

PMS, PREGNANCY and MENOPAUSE can all affect you emotionally.

DIETARY IMBALANCE

JUNK FOOD, OVEREATING, DIETING or a lack of certain NUTRIENTS can take their toll.

After all, FOOD is FUEL.

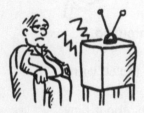

LACK OF EXERCISE

INACTIVITY can contribute greatly to a feeling of FLATNESS. Not only does your BODY run down, your MIND does too.

BURNOUT

OVERWORKING can mean little REST, POOR EATING HABITS and a flood of STRESS CHEMICALS.

PRESCRIPTION DRUGS

ALL drugs have SIDE-
EFFECTS — even over-
the-counter drugs such
as COLD PILLS, etc.

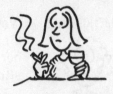

RECREATIONAL DRUGS

While drugs like ALCOHOL
may give you a temporary
lift, they will tend to
EXAGGERATE an existing
emotional state.

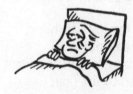

ILLNESS

SICKNESS, MEDICAL
PROCEDURE or MEDICATION
can mimic depression.
Naturally, CHRONIC,
DISABLING or TERMINAL
ILLNESS arouses deep
emotions.

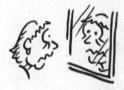

AGEING

Lack of general FITNESS,
the chronic effects of an
UNHEALTHY LIFESTYLE and
the EMOTIONAL changes of
AGEING can depress you.

 WORKING SOLUTIONS

☆ PMS — Keep a chart for several months to see if
there is a correlation between mood swings and
menstruation; if there is, PMS may be a problem.

☆ PREGNANCY — Your body goes through HUGE
changes during pregnancy and childbirth. BE
INFORMED, SEEK SUPPORT.

☆ MENOPAUSE

You may need to change your lifestyle and diet. You may need hormone replacement or natural alternatives. BECOME INFORMED.

☆ DIET

Would you expect your car to run efficiently on inferior or polluted fuel? It's the same for your body. BALANCE your diet — less FAT, more whole grain, vegies and fruit.

☆ EXERCISE

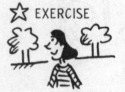

Simply walking for half an hour, three times a week not only increases your physical fitness, but has been proven to lift your spirits, too.

☆ BURNOUT

Is that PROMOTION, NEW TOY, or EXTRA MONEY more important than your LIFE?

Have a big think about your priorities.

☆ PRESCRIPTION
   DRUGS

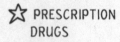

READ the literature. Find out what you are putting in your body.

☆ RECREATIONAL
   DRUGS

You know the dangers. Are you prepared to take the risks? Remember — too much of anything still ends up being TOO MUCH.

☆ ILLNESS

- Being AWARE of the effects of certain treatments and medications can prepare you for the symptoms.
Try to remain DETACHED.

- Coping with disability or serious illness can be difficult. ASK for support. TALK through your feelings.

☆ AGEING

You may need to REJUVENATE your life!

- Change your hairstyle.

- Refresh your wardrobe.

- Do something you've always wanted to do.

- You may need to RETHINK your philosophy — valuing things like WISDOM, INNER BEAUTY, LOVE and FREEDOM.

SOMETHING TO CHEW ON

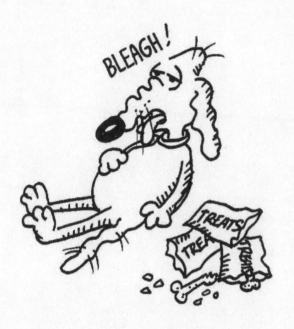

DIET AND DEPRESSION

What's in your FOOD BOWL?

Is it HEALTHY,
LIFE-ENHANCING
and MOOD-LIFTING?

Or is it HEAVY,
ENERGY-SAPPING
and a DOWNER?

Keeping an eye on your FOOD is one of the most important things you can do if you want to feel BETTER.

People either do not recognise or IGNORE the key role that FOOD plays in MOOD.

One of the TRAPS of depression is that your SELF-CARE takes a back seat, and your choice of FOOD when you're in a funk can often leave a lot to be desired.

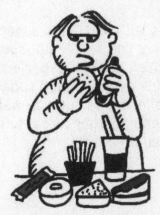

There will also be a tendency to go for what you might consider to be 'comfort food', such as heavy CARBS, FATS and SUGARS; but any 'comfort' to be derived from these in the short term can be COLD COMFORT in terms of your EMOTIONAL WELLBEING.

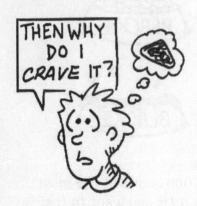

The reason that these foods are so compelling is that they are ADDICTIVE, as opposed to actually bringing you COMFORT.

The addictive element is SUGAR.

Whilst you may not necessarily have a SWEET TOOTH, processed and refined grains also convert to SUGAR in the body.

As with any DRUG, sugar will give you a HIGH; but soon after, you will experience a LOW as your blood sugar level drops and you will need another 'dose' to lift you up again.

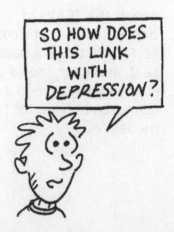

The *Whitehall Study* investigated the effects of sugar intake on mental health over 22 years, with test subjects being people who showed no signs of mental illness at the outset.

The link between high sugar consumption and the onset of depression became evident quite quickly and remained so throughout the study.

Sugar causes chemical changes and is linked to cellular inflammation, which is a likely contributor to depression.

At the very least, cutting down your sugar and carbohydrate intake is a move in the right direction.

You don't need to do anything complicated!

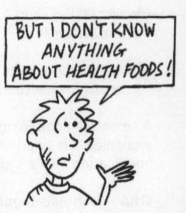

FOLLOW THESE GUIDELINES:

- ☆ Avoid any processed foods
- ☆ Increase your vegetables (not potatoes — they're starchy)
- ☆ Have 2 pieces of fruit a day
- ☆ Say 'yes' to good old meat and three veg
- ☆ Avoid takeaways
- ☆ Avoid cakes and sweets
- ☆ Fresh is best

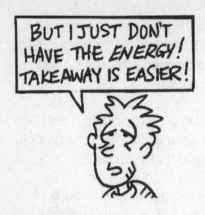

BUT I JUST DON'T HAVE THE *ENERGY*! TAKEAWAY IS EASIER!

Junk food SAPS a lot of your energy!

HOW HARD IS:

☆ Chopping up some vegies and steaming them while you grill a piece of steak or fish?

☆ Or making soup full of goodies and freezing it in batches?

☆ Or making an 'anti-depressant in a glass' — a healthy smoothie?

A smoothie containing some or all of the following ingredients is another (healthier) form of 'medication'. Here's why:

CHIA — contains tryptophan, which promotes production of serotonin — a natural anti-depressant.

BANANA — contains folic acid and vitamin B, which are often deficient in people with depression.

AVOCADO — contains potassium, which helps with mental fatigue.

BRAZIL NUTS — contain selenium, which helps fight free-radicals.

SPINACH — contains magnesium, which also increases serotonin.

OATS — are complex carbohydrates which help boost energy.

PUMPKIN SEEDS — contain zinc, which helps brain function.

Try this MOOD-BOOSTER SMOOTHIE

In a food processor, blend:
- 1 cup spinach
- ½ an avocado
- 1 tsp cinnamon (for flavour)
- 1 banana
- 1 tbsp pumpkin seeds
- 1 cup coconut water

You can add a little honey if you like.

Your food is either POISON or MEDICINE. It can make you SICK or WELL. It's THAT important!

OFF TO THE VETS

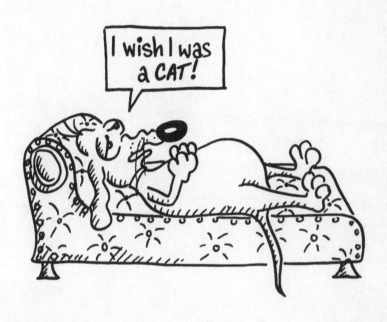

CHOOSING PROFESSIONAL HELP

Recruiting PROFESSIONAL HELP can be a valuable step in your journey out of depression, WHETHER or NOT you are making PROGRESS yourself.

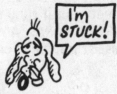

| IF YOU ARE NOT MAKING HEADWAY, A GOOD THERAPIST CAN: |

☆ BE A SOURCE OF EMPATHY, SUPPORT AND UNDERSTANDING

☆ CREATE A SAFE, NON-JUDGMENTAL ENVIRONMENT FOR YOU TO EXPRESS YOUR THOUGHTS AND FEELINGS

☆ BE A SOURCE OF MOTIVATION AND HOPE

☆ ASSIST YOU IN TAKING THE FIRST STEPS TO RECOVERY.

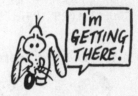

| IF YOU ARE MAKING PROGRESS, A GOOD THERAPIST CAN: |

☆ SUPPORT, ENCOURAGE AND STRENGTHEN YOUR PROGRESS

☆ PROVIDE DEEPER INSIGHTS INTO PATTERNS, STICKING POINTS, etc. FROM ANOTHER PERSPECTIVE

☆ SUPPORT YOU THROUGH TIMES OF SETBACK

☆ ASSIST YOU IN EXPLORING, UNDERSTANDING AND RELEASING THE PAST

☆ FORTIFY YOUR SELF-ESTEEM

☆ GUIDE YOU IN LIFE SKILLS, STRESS MANAGEMENT AND RELAXATION TECHNIQUES.

Who can help?

A trusted FRIEND, FAMILY MEMBER, SCHOOLMATE or WORK COLLEAGUE may provide the support you need; but if they can't, you may need a PROFESSIONAL. Among those who are TRAINED to assist people in crisis are:

SOCIAL WORKERS

DOCTORS

NURSES

PRIESTS OR MINISTERS OF RELIGION

CRISIS LINE COUNSELLORS

NATURAL PRACTITIONERS

> ALL OF THESE PEOPLE HAVE HAD, AS PART OF THEIR TRAINING, BASIC OR ADVANCED COUNSELLING, LISTENING SKILLS AND PROBLEM-SOLVING TECHNIQUES.

For DEEPER WORK, there are:

PROFESSIONAL COUNSELLORS
They provide all of the above, only to a more advanced level.

| TRAINING COURSE(S) |

PSYCHOLOGISTS
They explore the mental make-up of a person and how this causes certain behaviour.

| UNIVERSITY or POSTGRAD Degree or Diploma |

PSYCHIATRISTS
They examine the role of the SUBCONSCIOUS in relation to behaviour.

| MEDICAL DEGREE THEN SPECIALIST DEGREE IN MENTAL HEALTH |

PSYCHO-THERAPISTS
They employ specialised therapies (e.g. GESTALT, NLP, BODY WORK, etc.)

| TRAINING IN SPECIFIC FIELD(S) |

What to choose:

PSYCHIATRY tends to involve a long-term commitment with regular visits. It explores your childhood in depth. Psychiatrists can also prescribe medication.

PSYCHOLOGY can be short or long term. It will be more based in the present.

COUNSELLING involves active listening, understanding and non-intrusive guidance.

PSYCHOTHERAPY is a broad field, incorporating anything from quieter to more cathartic techniques. It can involve regular sessions or (for example) weekend intensives.

Who to choose:

The relationship between a therapist and client is a very intimate and special one.

In order to heal, you will be encouraged to express a lot of your hidden feelings, fears, hopes and dreams.

Therefore a therapist/client relationship should involve TRUST, UNDERSTANDING, HONESTY, SUPPORT, LACK OF JUDGMENT and SAFETY.

SO, SHOP AROUND!

Not all therapists, or indeed, therapies may suit you.

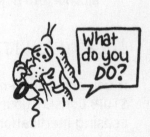

You have EVERY RIGHT to ask questions and explore options to make the best choice.

MEDICATION

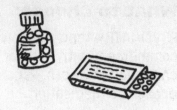

You can work through depression WITH drugs or WITHOUT.

In fact, even if untreated, depression will often eventually lift.

Your decision (and it is YOUR decision) to take medication if it is recommended by your GP or therapist is best made only if you are fully informed.

QUESTIONS TO ASK

☆ WHAT WILL THE MEDICATION DO?

☆ WHAT ARE THE SIDE EFFECTS?

☆ HOW LONG BEFORE THE MEDICATION TAKES EFFECT? (Some anti-depressants take time to take effect.)

☆ WHAT IS INVOLVED IN COMING OFF THE MEDICATION?

☆ WHAT ARE THE OTHER OPTIONS?

☆ ARE THERE ANY PRECAUTIONS (e.g. certain foods, alcohol, etc.)?

IMPORTANT!

If you are taking medication, DO NOT SUDDENLY STOP! Consult your doctor or therapist before ceasing medication. You may need to be WEANED off the drug slowly.

CHOOSING THE DRUG-FREE OPTION

You may wish to work through your depression WITHOUT medication.

If so, you will need to:

☆ IDENTIFY THE FACTORS IN YOUR LIFE THAT HAVE CONTRIBUTED TO YOUR DEPRESSION

☆ RE-EVALUATE, CHANGE OR REMOVE AS MANY OF THESE AS POSSIBLE

☆ BE PREPARED TO MAKE RECOVERY A PRIORITY OVER COMFORT FOR A WHILE

☆ BE PREPARED TO RISK REJECTION, LACK OF SECURITY, etc. WHILE YOU MAKE CHANGES

☆ BECOME WELL INFORMED ABOUT DEPRESSION, PERSONAL DEVELOPMENT, etc. (THIS BOOK SHOULD HELP!)

☆ BE VERY TRUTHFUL WITH YOURSELF AND OTHERS ABOUT PATTERNS, ISSUES, etc.

☆ BE OPEN ABOUT YOUR FEELINGS, NEEDS, etc.

☆ SET GOALS FOR YOURSELF (AND REWARDS FOR ACHIEVING THEM!).

YOU MAY NEED MEDICATION IF:

☆ YOU ARE OVERWHELMED TO THE POINT OF IMMOBILITY

☆ YOUR DEPRESSION IS CLEARLY OF A BIOLOGICAL NATURE

☆ YOUR MOOD SWINGS ARE EXTREME

☆ YOU NEED 'TIME OUT' FROM YOUR DISTRESS IN ORDER TO GAIN A BETTER PERSPECTIVE.

For deep or persistant depression, MEDICATION combined with THERAPY may be the best option.

The reason for this is that while MEDICATION may provide PHYSICAL RELIEF, the PSYCHOLOGICAL or LIFESTYLE FACTORS that have contributed to your depression will need to be addressed for there to be LONG-TERM IMPROVEMENT.

Think of it THIS WAY

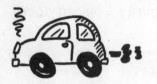

Say your CAR is running low on OIL

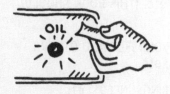

MEDICATION may work in a similar way as covering over the WARNING LIGHT ...

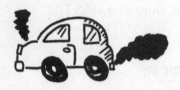

... but sooner or later, you're going to need to attend to that OIL if you want your car to run well!

MEDICATION is best seen as a TEMPORARY option, to give you some SPACE and DISTANCE from the problem, so that you may view it more OBJECTIVELY and attend to what you need to.

Finally ...

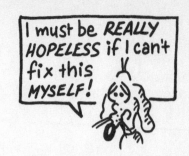

Seeking help is NOT a sign of WEAKNESS or FAILURE!

You got into this situation because, up till now, you did not KNOW the life skills that would prevent this from occurring.

In fact, it is a STRONG person who acknowledges and expresses their vulnerability to another and a truly COURAGEOUS person who is prepared to honestly face and CHANGE the elements in his/her life that are not working well.

Now and then, we ALL need help.

☆ If your PIPES are leaking, you call a PLUMBER!

☆ If your WIRES are shorting, you call an ELECTRICIAN!

☆ If you can't work your COMPUTER, you'd ask an IT TECHNICIAN/SPECIALIST to help you!

Human beings are COMPLEX creatures.

Sometimes we get so stuck in ourselves we need someone else to provide another view.

NO SHAME IN THAT!

THE BLACK DOG AND THE BLACK HOLE

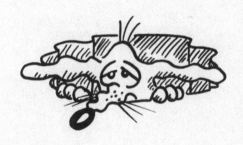

WHEN THERE SEEMS NO HOPE AND NO POINT

No book dealing with the subject of depression can overlook the kind of despair that leads to suicidal thoughts or even suicide attempts.

This is indeed, a common aspect of depression. You can reach a point where you feel ...

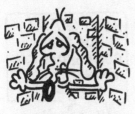

SO STUCK THAT THERE SEEMS NO WAY OUT

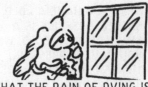

THAT THE PAIN OF DYING IS BRIEF, AND THE PAIN OF LIVING GOES ON AND ON

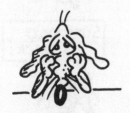

SO ALONE AND UNLOVED THAT YOUR LEAVING WOULD BE NO BIG DEAL

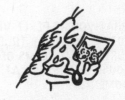

THAT YOU ARE JUST A BURDEN ON OTHERS AND THEY'D BE BETTER OFF WITHOUT YOU

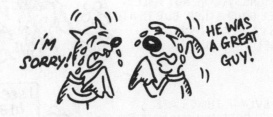

THAT THOSE WHO HURT YOU MIGHT FINALLY UNDERSTAND THE SUFFERING THEY CAUSED YOU IF YOU CHECKED OUT!

While reaching such a state indicates that you are, indeed, suffering a great deal, the REALITY may not be what you think!

Let's take a look —

1. WHEN YOU HAVE A COLD, YOU SNEEZE. SNEEZING IS A SYMPTOM OF A COLD. WHEN YOU HAVE DEPRESSION, THINGS LOOK BLEAK. IT'S A SYMPTOM OF DEPRESSION. YOUR DEPRESSION IS THE REAL PROBLEM, NOT YOUR LIFE!

Hey, I GET IT! Things aren't SUPPOSED to look BRIGHT if you're DEPRESSED!

2. WHAT YOU'RE PERCEIVING IS NOT NECESSARILY TRUE. IT'S JUST HOW IT SEEMS BECAUSE YOU'RE DEPRESSED AT THE MOMENT.

Sure looks BLACK!

3. THE THINGS IN YOUR LIFE ARE BEING COLOURED BY YOUR EMOTIONS. YOU'RE NOT ABLE TO SEE GOOD STUFF, BUT THAT DOESN'T MEAN IT'S NOT THERE!

I see NOTHING GOOD!

4. AND EVEN IF THINGS ARE PRETTY ROTTEN, YOU'LL HAVE A BETTER CHANCE OF DEALING WITH THEM IF YOU GET YOUR DEPRESSION SORTED!

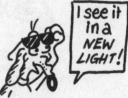

I see it in a NEW LIGHT!

VITAL POINT:

It's not a good idea to make a PERMANENT DECISION based on a TEMPORARY EMOTIONAL STATE! (Even if it's dragged on for a while).

And death is VERY VERY permanent!

At this point, death may seem like an attractive concept — even a little ROMANTIC.

But it's important that you really GET IT — DEAD IS DEAD.

There's no half-dead or 'I'll give it a go' dead. Dead is FINAL.

Mostly, when people reach this point, they don't so much want to die but crave REST, RELIEF or RESCUE.

And usually, it is in the wee, small hours that this 'solution' seems most compelling.

RULE NUMBER 1 — WAIT UNTIL MORNING!

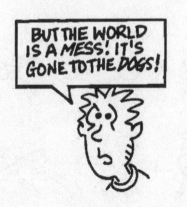

Firstly, that's an OPINION that you currently hold.

Opinions become BELIEFS when we invest in them often enough.

But beliefs are still just OPINIONS. They are not FACTS.

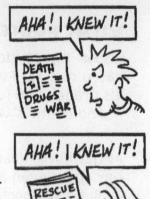

When you have a belief about something, you look for EVIDENCE.

And yes, you will find evidence ...

... but so will someone who has a different opinion from you!

So how is getting all MESSED UP about the state of things going to IMPROVE those things?

Does feeling bad about something actually HELP anything?

We all contribute to the way the world works — every single day. If you really think you have no influence, THINK AGAIN! The flavour of one single encounter can affect THOUSANDS!

YOU make that difference! You MATTER!

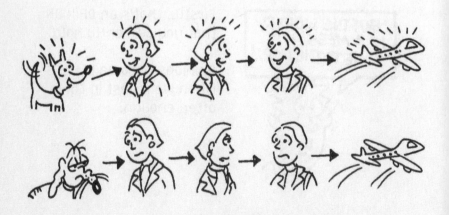

It is NOT your time. It is NOT in your script.
Yes, you feel like absolute crap at the moment
and maybe you have for some time; but how long
you continue to feel this way is a choice you CAN
make, using the tools in this book.

Make that choice. As soon as you can.

Feeling better is there. It exists. You just need to
reach out for it.

ASK YOURSELF —

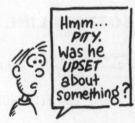

☆ Have I REALLY explored ALL
of my options, sought the
RIGHT HELP, WORKED on my
problems?

☆ What would be the REAL
impact of my death on others
(not the fantasised one)?

☆ Is there REALLY no hope, or
have I just lost sight of it?

☆ If nobody CARES, have I given
them a CHANCE to? Have I
told them how I REALLY feel?
Have I asked for help in a
CLEAR and DIRECT way?

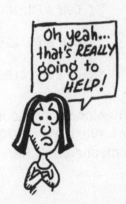

☆ If the ones I love were
SUFFERING, would I want
them to DIE to ease *my*
burden?

If you are still considering this decision, then know that you are not WELL ENOUGH to make such a big DECISION!

You''re not yourself, are you?

You're not thinking straight, are you?

You're not really in the best position to make a SENSIBLE CHOICE, are you?

If you were going to make any other MONUMENTAL decision in your life, you'd seek EXPERT ADVICE, wouldn't you?

Well, there are few more monumental decisions than this one. You need a SECOND OPINION.

BOTTOM LINE —

TELL SOMEONE! ASK FOR HELP!

☆ Call TELEPHONE COUNSELLING

☆ Call a FRIEND

☆ Call a FAMILY MEMBER

☆ Call a TEACHER, MINISTER, COUNSELLOR

When choosing your confidante, keep in mind that not everyone's GOOD at it! Don't be disheartened if someone can't handle it; the important thing is that you have reached out! Keep reaching out until you get the help you need. This is why a professional is often the best choice.

Think again.
Hang on.

☆ You may have lost HOPE, but there's always the HOPE of finding HOPE.

☆ You don't know what's next in the script! You're just stuck in the DRAMA! Read on — the NEXT PAGES could be ...

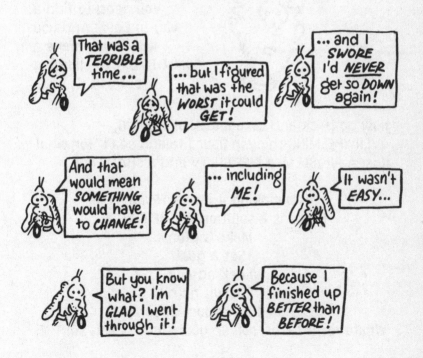

SUICIDE IS NOT FOR YOU. It's just not.
NOTHING is WORTH IT. Forget it. It's just a BAD IDEA.
And understand this: Life is DIFFICULT. It is for
EVERYONE.
The art is in RISING ABOVE, BECOMING STRONGER,
LEARNING FROM MISTAKES, BEING RESILIENT.
You're BIGGER than this. You just forgot that you
are.

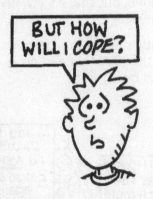

You'll cope because
that's what you need
to do now.

You need to find a
way to COPE. And you
will, if you make a
COMMITMENT to climbing
out of this hole.

Now go back and take a look at this BIG,
OVERWHELMING thing in your life and see it for what
it is: A PROBLEM, a DIFFICULTY and a CHALLENGE.

Stop making it into a TRAGEDY.
There is a solution to EVERYTHING.
Make a plan
Set a goal
Seek advice
Recruit help
Join a support group
Whatever it takes, roll up your sleeves and SORT IT.

Then it goes away.

15

NEW TRICKS

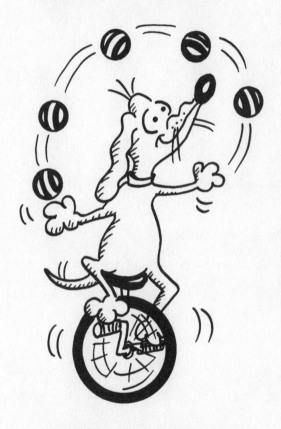

KEEPING RECOVERY ON TRACK

There's on old saying —
'YOU CAN'T TEACH AN OLD
DOG NEW TRICKS!' Well,
since CAN'T is one of
those negative, limiting
words that you're
learning to avoid,
(along with 'SHOULD' etc.)
We'll swap it for —

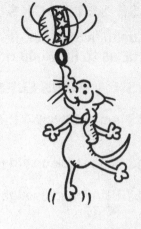

'YOU <u>CAN</u> TEACH AN OLD
DOG NEW TRICKS —
IT MIGHT JUST TAKE A BIT
LONGER!'

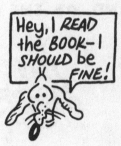

And, learning any new
skill involves TIME,
PATIENCE, PERSEVERENCE
and LEARNING FROM
MISTAKES!

Changing a LIFETIME of
PATTERNS is going to
require a FOCUSED EFFORT over a PERIOD OF TIME.

For a while, as is true when trying anything
new, it may feel a bit uncomfortable, silly, or
unnatural to be CHECKING IN ON YOURSELF and
CORRECTING yourself all the time.

And now and then —

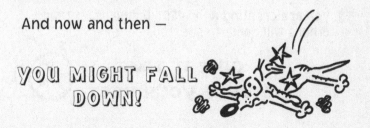

YOU MIGHT FALL
DOWN!

USE SETBACKS AS A TOOL

Usually, a SETBACK is going to give you a VITAL CLUE as to HOW you got stuck and HOW to PROCEED.

ASK YOURSELF:

☆ Am I RERUNNING the past?

☆ Am I stuck on old HURT?

☆ Have I had enough REST?

☆ Am I in a RUT?

☆ What needs my ATTENTION?

☆ What am I TELLING myself?

AND, AS THE OLD SONG GOES:

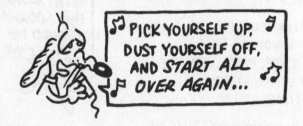

♫ PICK YOURSELF UP, DUST YOURSELF OFF, AND *START ALL OVER AGAIN...* ♫

This may feel like a DRAG, but remember ...

☆ Each small VICTORY adds up to SUCCESS

☆ You are STRENGTHENING yourself against having to ever REPEAT this again

☆ You are LEARNING! You are gaining WISDOM

☆ You are creating a RESPECT for yourself that others will come to see, too.

GIVE IT TIME
GIVE IT YOUR BEST

Moving on means LETTING GO of:

☆ THINGS THAT NO LONGER SERVE YOU

☆ PEOPLE WHO BRING YOU DOWN

☆ AN ATTACHMENT TO SUFFERING

☆ SEEKING AFFIRMATION OF YOUR WORTH FROM OTHER THAN YOURSELF

☆ OLD 'STORIES' THAT DEPRESS YOU

☆ AN IDEA THAT YOU ARE POWERLESS

☆ JUNK FROM THE PAST.

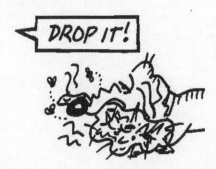

Why on earth are you hanging on to SUFFERING and STRUGGLE?

You don't want to be depressed, so choose NOT to be! You could actually be having FUN instead!

And yes, you do have that choice. It's a DECISION — a decision you may need to make again and again, especially when tough challenges come your way, as they WILL.

16

GOOD DOG!

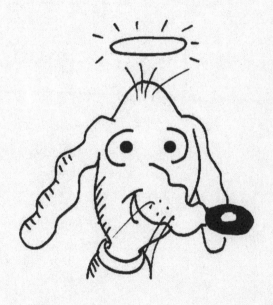

THE FOUR KEYS TO FREEDOM

There are four keys to get out of this prison:

FORGIVENESS

GRATITUDE

LOVE

and GIVING

1.
FORGIVENESS

Don't you want to be
FORGIVEN when you
MESS UP?

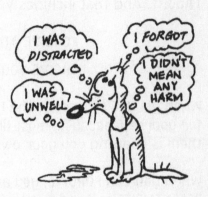

So does EVERYONE!

But being forgiven is unlikely if YOU can't
forgive someone else or yourself!

The UNFORGIVING MIND is in turmoil because it:

- SEES THE WORST
- EXPECTS THE WORST — AND GETS IT
- SEES 'CRIMES' OR 'SINS' INSTEAD OF MISTAKES
- HOLDS ON TO HURTS AND SLIGHTS
- CAN'T TRUST

FORGIVENESS is learned; it's not innate. It means choosing to let go of any anger, hurt or resentment that weighs YOU down. It means cutting the emotional ties that keep you bound to the past or to someone else.

It also means seeing that EVERYONE makes mistakes and can only do the best with what they HAVE, what they KNOW and what they have been TAUGHT. And that includes YOU.

FORGIVE OTHERS

FORGIVE YOURSELF

When you let others off the hook, you do the same for yourself because, most likely, what you see in them is showing you your own SHORTFALLS.

When you can FORGIVE, you are FREE — of SHAME, RESENTMENT and the burden of carrying around someone else with you.

2. GRATITUDE

When you're depressed you think you're BADLY OFF. Gratitude says you're NOT.

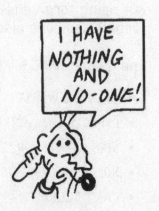

I HAVE NOTHING AND NO-ONE!

When you're depressed, all your focus is on what is MISSING, rather than what you HAVE.

Do you have FOOD in your BELLY?
Be GRATEFUL.

A ROOF over your HEAD?
Be GRATEFUL.

MONEY (at least enough to buy this book!)?
Be GRATEFUL.

FAMILY? FRIENDS? A PET? SUNSHINE? TREES?
BE GRATEFUL.

No matter how small or meagre, you have SOMETHING to be grateful for. Do not take this for GRANTED. These things are GIFTS.

3. LOVE

There's a guaranteed way to get love and that is to GIVE it — UNCONDITIONALLY.

Unconditionally means just that — NO CONDITIONS!

Not 'I'll love you as long as you please me'
    'I'll love you only if you love me back'
    'I'll love you if you give me something'

Love SOMETHING — anything!

A DOG, a CAT, DRAWING, CROSSWORDS PUZZLES, ROCKS, ANTS — it doesn't matter what — LOVE it.

Then love YOURSELF, because when you do, you

- Won't take any CRAP
- Will take PRIDE in yourself
- Will look after yourself
- Will VALUE yourself; regardless of what anyone else says or does.

When you LOVE YOURSELF:

- If things go pear-shaped, you set it RIGHT so that you feel BETTER
- If you lose something or someone, you look for the OPPORTUNITY this brings
- If someone is NASTY to you, you PITY them their mean spirit and recognse their FEAR.

4. GIVING

We can all get a bit caught up in OURSELVES, especially when we're stuck in emotional pain.

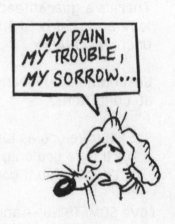

MY PAIN, MY TROUBLE, MY SORROW...

Giving to others can show you that:

- You're not ALONE
- We're all in this TOGETHER
- Your struggle is not the ONLY kind of struggle
- Looking beyond yourself is a way out of yourself
- Lifting others lifts you.

And — everything you GIVE comes back to you. Think on this. What are you giving? What are you getting?

If you want LOVE, give it.
If you want SUPPORT, give it.
If you want FRIENDS, be friendly.
If you want to feel BETTER,
help someone else feel better.

In the end, you are giving to YOURSELF. True giving is SELFLESS. It expects nothing in return. That's the tricky part. Give simply because it feels GOOD to do so. The rest will follow.

Giving can be as simple as smiling at a passer-by or being generous with your compliments on social media.

Best of all, when you FORGIVE, are GRATEFUL, LOVING and GIVING, these things start to COME BACK TO YOU!

THAT'S how you change the world!

Okay, it's time to move on.

There's a LIFE out there to which you are every bit as entitled as anyone else on this planet! Start ENJOYING it instead of using your precious time and energy on all this dark stuff.

Darkness is only ONE HALF of the story and you've explored it enough now. Time to explore the LIGHT.

There is only one thing left to do:

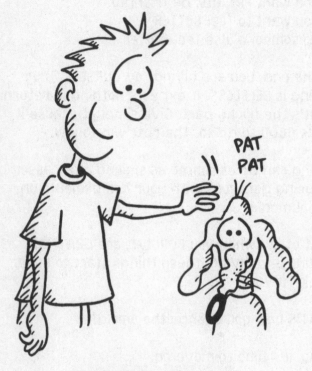

PAT PAT

HEAL